The Necklace

Rave Reviews for The Necklace

For many couples, surviving a miscarriage, the loss of a child, or endless infertility battles can be emotionally devastating. But God! *The Necklace* gives the reader an intimate look inside the real-life struggles of women (and men) who've experienced this unimaginable pain. In every case, it was their unshakable Faith in God, the hope of the tiny mustard seed, and the support of their "sisterhood" that carried them through!

—Dr. Tim Clinton, LPC, LMFT, BCPCC - President American Association of Christian Counselors

The Necklace is like chicken soup for the soul meets sisterhood of the traveling pants! Infertility is no walk in the park and this book will be there for you. If you or someone you know is struggling with infertility or loss this is a must have book! It will encourage you, increase your faith and give you the strength you need to never give up!

—Coffey & Criscilla Anderson
Stars of Country Ever After

Holy Love is the essence of God, who before creation existed in perfect triune harmony. But there was a divine yearning for children, and it became manifest when God created humankind in His image. The Lord imprinted that divine desire for children into the DNA of our hearts, and if impeded, unfulfilled or lost, it can feel like a spiritual disconnect as lonely as Christ was on the cross. Nicole Wood courageously shares her journey through infertility, loss and the isolation of putting on a smile to cover silent pain. This book will infuse courage into women on similar paths and the husbands who walk with them hand in hand. When you read this book, you will feel like Nicole is personally ministering to you. I believe you will receive healing and a new portion of faith, hope and love.

—**Rev. Daniel E. Kennedy**, MC, Marriage & Family Therapy, Chief Executive Officer, Oasis of Hope Hospital

The Necklace is an amazing collection of powerful testimonies from women who have walked the difficult road of infertility. Though their experiences are different, each of them leaned on God to provide strength, trusting Him in the midst of questions, difficulty, heartbreak, hope, and joy. You'll be inspired and encouraged through the stories of these amazing women, as well as through the beautiful grace and comfort that the Lord offered them in the midst of their journeys.

—**Dr. Sam Chand**, Leadership consultant and best-selling author

As an oncologist, many of my patients have questions about fertility or share how infertility has affected their emotional health. I need to connect patients to resources that improve health and foster hope. *The Necklace* is an incredible resource I will be sharing with my patients. I highly recommend you read this hope-building book.

–**Francisco Contreras**, MD
President & Chair, Oasis of Hope Hospital
www.OasisofHope.com

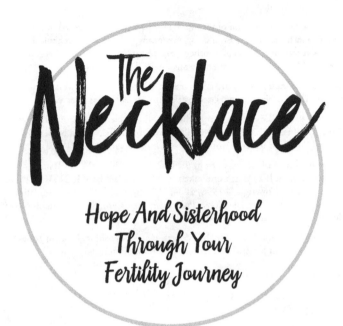

The Necklace

Hope And Sisterhood
Through Your
Fertility Journey

Nicole Wood

NEW YORK

LONDON • NASHVILLE • MELBOURNE • VANCOUVER

The Necklace

Hope and Sisterhood Through Your Fertility Journey

Published in New York, New York, by Morgan James Publishing. Morgan James is a trademark of Morgan James, LLC. www.MorganJamesPublishing.com

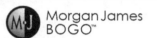

Morgan James BOGO™

A **FREE** ebook edition is available for you or a friend with the purchase of this print book.

CLEARLY SIGN YOUR NAME ABOVE

Instructions to claim your free ebook edition:
1. Visit MorganJamesBOGO.com
2. Sign your name CLEARLY in the space above
3. Complete the form and submit a photo of this entire page
4. You or your friend can download the ebook to your preferred device

ISBN 9781631954672 paperback
ISBN 9781631954689 ebook
Library of Congress Control Number: 2021932202

Cover and Interior Design by:
Chris Treccani
www.3dogcreative.net

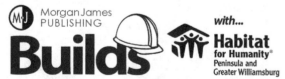

Morgan James PUBLISHING

Builds

with...

Habitat for Humanity®
Peninsula and Greater Williamsburg

Morgan James is a proud partner of Habitat for Humanity Peninsula and Greater Williamsburg. Partners in building since 2006.

Get involved today! Visit
MorganJamesPublishing.com/giving-back

For all those facing infertility, loss,
and everything in-between.

Contents

Acknowledgments

Words can't express the magnitude of my gratitude to my Lord and Savior, Jesus Christ. Thank You for inspiring this Sisterhood of women, myself included. Your words and promises are healing reminders of Your faithfulness and goodness.

To my precious family, particularly my husband, Joe, and all my sisters featured in *The Necklace*, thank you for your support, vulnerability, and hearts toward God. Your faith encourages me and is a huge part of this book. There is no book without each of you.

Thank you to Morgan James Publishing, the entire team, for believing in this book and taking it global.

And thank you to the Sisterhood of women all over the world, those who've already worn the mustard seed necklace and those who are yet to feel its power, to those struggling with loss or infertility or both . . . know you are loved.

Foreword

I had it all figured out and I had a plan. I'd been married five years, and now, I was going to get pregnant at age thirty . . .

Boom!

Right on schedule!

Then, just as we were making all our preparations, I found out I had stage four cervical cancer. (So much for my plans.)

Years later, we finally conceived. But, just three-and-a-half months later, a crushing miscarriage and the excruciating task of telling everyone we'd lost our baby followed. Emptiness, guilt, and unfathomable despair!

There are many couples out there that have been hoping, praying, and trying for so much longer. They've been picking up the pieces of their broken hearts, putting on brave faces, pretending to go on with their daily routines (as if any of it really mattered), and just holding it all together for . . . one . . . more . . . day!

I'm so thankful to have this book as such a valuable resource and for Nicole Wood, who so bravely brings to light the devastating hurt that a lot of women (and men) painfully struggle to keep hidden. In doing so, she has made herself vulnerable by opening up her heart to us and sharing her own deeply personal experiences, anxieties, thoughts, and fears.

This book is filled with unimaginable, heart wrenching stories of loss—but more importantly, unwavering faith in God and the hope and strength to keep going, even when nothing seems to be going as we planned.

Is that you? Did you feel like you were the only one? I did.

Infertility, surrogacy, fostered, or adopted—I don't know what I would've done without the dear man who adopted me when I was three—motherhood can take so many different paths. And all of them, in God's perfect plan, in His perfect timing, not ours!

The Necklace is a precious collection of individual stories and experiences of women connected by a spirit of HOPE, inspired by the amazing mustard seed necklace. It will remind you that many of us share the same thoughts, fears, and insecurities. But if we can manage to muster just that tiny seed of faith, God's goodness and faithfulness toward us is unshakeable!

This is a book worthy of sharing with all your sisters.

I love how Nicole sums it up: "We do not always have the answers, but we have each other, and we have hope."

Through it all, we are your sisterhood—standing strong with you. You are not alone!

—Nicole Crank, Host of *The Nicole Crank Show*, author, speaker, pastor, & co-founder of FaithChurch.com

Introduction

One in eight couples struggles with infertility.

Infertility is the inability to conceive a child, clinically described as: a disease of the reproductive system defined by the failure to achieve a clinical pregnancy after twelve months of trying to conceive.

It is such a widespread issue yet so lonely.

The journey of infertility is one that affects each person and family differently, yet the heartache appears to be so much the same. There is such a collective bond between those whom are affected by infertility and fertility issues. Many couples proceed with in vitro fertilization—otherwise known as IVF—adoption, or surrogacy. All are incredibly intense, expensive, and challenging, forcing many to face unexpected and complex journeys to grow their families.

The Necklace is a powerful and true story of a mustard seed necklace that was passed from woman to woman though their fertility journey. Each unique story tugs at the heart strings yet provides encouragement and comfort for all in knowing they are not alone. With faith, all things are possible.

No matter what the individual journey is, *The Necklace* shares true stories of women and their families that have faced it *all* and made it through to the other side. It provides a community—a Sisterhood of women who know exactly what it feels like to hear the unthinkable, feel the unimaginable, and still one day, finally see the light at the end of the tunnel.

There is such a need to connect those on their fertility/infertility journeys, and this book makes it a possibility. Through reading each true story, the relevant and practical advice from others who have been there, Scripture, prayers, and the encouraging thoughts within, the reader will not be disappointed. They will be longing for more.

Come, take the journey with us and find out how the necklace took on a life of its own and changed the world, one woman at a time! It is my honor and privilege to introduce you to some of the strongest most courageous women I have ever met.

Never lose your faith: with God all things are possible!

1

Meet Me, Nicole

The Journey Begins

As I stood before my incredible husband Joe, then jumped up and down with exhilaration, my mind not able to catch up with my heart! I remember it as if it was yesterday, standing there holding our positive pregnancy test. There had been times I never thought that day would come.

I married the man of my dreams one month after my twenty-sixth birthday. We were drawn to each other like magnets, life partners ready and willing to take on the world. We had discussed having kids even while we were dating, and I was always on board about it being the "right time." Joe, however, had taken a little time to catch the vision. After we got married, we wanted to spend time with each other building the right foundation for our marriage, traveling, having fun, being newlyweds, and spending quality time with Joe's two young children—my new, beautiful bonus children.

This seemed like the perfect plan and after being married for five incredible years, we decided it was time to start growing our family. Of course, I knew it might take time to get pregnant, but I had no idea that fertility had a stopwatch on it. Fertility age became a new reality for me as I started my research. Did you know that a woman who is pregnant at the age of thirty-five is considered to be at an advanced maternal age (previously referred to as geriatric pregnancy)? *Say what? Geriatric?*

That, to me, was absolutely crazy. At age thirty-one, I thought, "Oh boy, where does this leave us?" And so the pressure began: if we wanted to have more than one child we had to hurry up and get pregnant with the first one before we ran out of time to have our second, or possibly third one. Now, to some people this may sound silly, but to countless others, I know you are all nodding your heads in agreement.

You see, as women, we are all on this fertility journey together; actually, I like to call it a Sisterhood. We have different stories, feelings, emotions, and realities, but we are intertwined in a special way. As woman, we experience something that's almost impossible to put into words, but we can all feel it. Whether you have perfect reproductive health or you are struggling with the upward battle of infertility, we are all sisters. Yes sisters—our hearts rage with excitement when family and friends get pregnant and our hearts are broken to pieces and hurting with those who are struggling with fertility or the unthinkable, the loss of a child. As women we share a bond that is pretty phenomenal.

Whether you realize it or not, you are not alone on your journey, and no matter what, there is always hope. Do not give up.

I can say this because I have experienced firsthand the journey of the necklace, a beautiful mustard seed necklace that has taken on a life of its own. I consider myself a woman of faith; it defines who I am and how I live my life. With that being said, I much prefer listening to talking. Being a counselor is my passion, so I come by this honestly. My faith is not something I ever push on anyone but am always ready and willing to share.

When I bought the necklace, I wore it every single day as a visual and tangible reminder to keep my faith, no matter what we faced on our fertility journey. The necklace holds a tiny mustard seed, which reminded me of one of my favorite Scriptures.

Matthew 17:20: *So Jesus said to them, "Because of your unbelief; for assuredly, I say to you, if you have faith as a mustard*

*seed, you will say to this mountain, 'Move from here to there,'
and it will move, and nothing will be impossible for you."*

Being in the Sisterhood, you know how important it is to keep the faith when you are facing the unknown, another negative pregnancy test, IVF treatments, adoption meetings, surrogacy, devastating loss, and everything in-between that comes our way in life.

As Joe and I were trying to conceive, I said to him, "Babe, if it's not this month then maybe we need to go in for fertility testing to see where we are at." When month six of a negative pregnancy test rolled around, I must admit, my faith was dwindling. Now, please don't get mad at me; I know six months is not a long time, especially compared to so many of those I love who have tried six, seven, even eight years—yes, years! But to me, six months felt like forever because I knew my maternal clock was ticking. I felt as if I was racing against time.

In month seven, I was jumping up and down with tears of joy streaming down my face, and I knew I would never forget that feeling. I would never forget the way my heart felt or the look on my husband's lovable face.

I continued to wear my necklace through my pregnancy because I faced more than I was prepared for. In the first trimester, I started bleeding and called the nurse immediately. She shared with me that I could be having a miscarriage and to simply rest. Sisterhood, how do we rest at a time like this?

For me, there was only one answer: you rest in HIM. Looking at the necklace around my neck and seeing that seed was symbolic for me. The tiny seed in the necklace and the tiny seed in my womb would be forever intertwined. I chose every day to never lose my faith, no matter what I faced. To cherish hope.

Now, this is much easier said than done, right? As I have stood with family members and friends, crying out, "Why me, why us, why my baby, why God, whhhhhy?" These moments are heartbreaking and devastating to say the least. We do not always have the answers, but we have each other, and we have hope.

Praying and waiting is what we did. We believed for the best, tried not to worry or let our minds wander, and then we put the rest in God's hands. I knew He was with us, and I could feel His presence inside me. He was the "light unto my path" of faith, one that felt a bit dark during that time.

Thankfully, nine months later, I gave birth to our son. We named him Corban Ryker. Corban means *belonging to God*. Ryker means *powerful ruler*.

You see, my story with the necklace was not over yet. When Corban was born, the doctors were concerned because he was not crying. I prayed and called out to God for help. I closed my eyes, and it was as if no one else was in the room. I was not going to accept their words of fear. I heard the nurse say, "Whatever you are doing, keep doing it; it's working!" Corban ended up in the Neonatal Intensive Care Unit. Anyone that has ever had a child in the NICU knows how daunting it can feel.

Less than twenty-four hours after I had given birth, a flood of nurses and doctors came into our room, said a ton of things, and then swept him away. Our precious baby boy . . . taken away from us in a matter of minutes. I stared at Joe in disbelief, shocked and listless.

Of course, they were an incredible team of doctors and nurses, fighting to save Corban's life, but everything was a blur to me, including reality. I had just delivered my son, and then he was taken away and placed in a special room where you had to wear unique protective suits, masks, and gloves. They had no idea what was wrong with him, but they knew they had to figure it out quickly. My mind never stopped racing, and I don't think I ever stopped crying or praying. Again, I needed my reminder—the necklace. My faith! Do not give up, do not lose hope, keep praying. *Nothing is impossible with God.*

Thankfully, a nurse discovered an abnormality in Corban's mouth, which led them to do further testing. They discovered he had a severe infection. To this day, they do not know what it was. As Corban now says, "It's a mystery!"

We do know that for eight days of our lives, it felt like time stood still, and I slowly suffocated under the weight of the unknown. I felt helpless, beyond worried. The little tubes in his head and arms seemed like lifelines straight to my heart. Constantly tugging at me. Sisterhood, you know what I mean. My baby was lying there, all wrapped up, without me. How do I move forward without him in my arms? I faced two choices. I could live in fear and give up hope, or I could keep praying and stand strong in my faith.

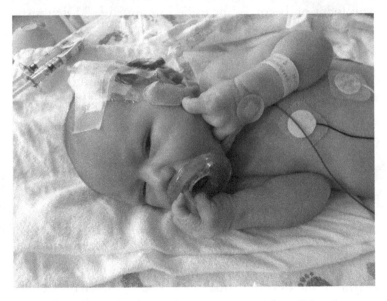

Of course, the latter became my reality. The doctors warned us that Corban needed to gain weight by this day or told us the medicine had to do this, by that time. It seemed every day, a new goal emerged for him to achieve! But through each answered prayer, my faith grew stronger . . . and so did Corban. Joe, next to God, of course, was my pillar of strength. We were there for each other, side-by-side, ready to battle for our son. We quietly played our worship music and sang in the NICU, yearning for an atmosphere of miracles. The medical staff asked us to turn our music down a bit. Of course, we did and offered our apologies. We just knew that we wanted Corban and his other tiny friends to be surrounded by peace and joy rather than alarms and beeps. We always say, "Whatever you focus on becomes magnified in your life." Obviously, Corban's healing was our focus.

When we finally got the news we could go home with our son, I was beyond excited yet scared beyond measure. We were responsible for this helpless, beautiful baby, one who had an entire team of doctors taking care of him night and day. What if we made a mistake or we didn't know what to do? A whole new set of fears set in; Sisterhood, are you with me? Babies don't come with user manuals! How were we going to take care of this precious baby boy?

Where's my necklace?

One of our favorite nurses said, "You will just muddle through one day at a time." She was right. That's exactly what we did. We endured a time in our lives, which we were not prepared for, but it was quite apparent that God was. He was there with us every step of the way (and still is) as we faced this new challenge in our lives.

One day, months after Corban was born, we strode through church and a powerful song echoed through the hallways, it's lyrics so bold my body became covered with goosebumps! I was wearing my necklace, and it was at that exact moment, I knew it was time. A still, small voice inside me knew that one of my "sisters" needed this necklace.

The song spoke of the great unknowns and where our feet might fail, there is mystery; yet, our faith will survive. I knew we had so much mystery ahead of us, but no matter what, our faith would stand—as it did through the challenges, obstacles and spiritual attacks we faced when our beautiful daughter, Isabella Grace, was born on August 14, 2015. But I am getting ahead of myself. That is a story for another time.

OK, Sisterhood, back to the song: as the church worshipped in the background, I knew it was time. Time to obey that still small voice, which I knew as God, telling me to pass the necklace on.

I asked my friend, Terrina, if I could speak with her. She and her husband had been trying for many years to conceive. I said, "I have worn this necklace through my journey with Corban, and now it's time for you to wear it on your journey." With tears in her eyes, she gave me the biggest hug and asked me to put the necklace on her.

Then and there, we knew we'd be forever interwoven by faith, hope, and the mustard seed. The Sisterhood and the journey of the necklace were only just beginning.

****

I should have known better than to believe my part of this incredible journey was over. As the pages of this beautiful book were coming together, the stories of our lives continued to blossom. Recently, my family and I decided to make a couple of big moves across the country to be a part of an incredible church, and along our journey, there were many surprises, including me jumping up and down again while holding a positive pregnancy test! That's right! At thirty-eight years old, unexpectedly, God blessed us with another precious gift!

My husband and I were elated and just knew that God was up to something really big! Teasing my husband about his age was the best part! Our special surprise came on the month of both of our birthdays! Of course, we started planning doctor's appointments, thinking of baby names, and everything in-between. As time went on, we decided to tell Corban and Bella they were going to have a baby brother or sister. The joy on their faces was completely indescribable! Kids in a candy store does not even come close.

They were instantly in love, so when the time came to tell them their baby sibling had gone to heaven to be with Jesus, the devastation was gut wrenching. Watching my babies grieve broke my heart in a way I could have never imagined possible. Consoling them with giant tears running down their faces brought my husband and I to our knees. Both physically and spiritually.

We had fallen in love with our precious gift the moment we heard the little heartbeat and saw the tiny outline in my belly. Typing these words still feels surreal, and honestly, I replay the events that occurred over and over, like a movie in my head.

What stands out the most is the moment I fell to my knees in the shower, praying and crying out to God. I had been bleeding and gone to the doctor for some answers, and although my doctor had some concerns, she was still hopeful. Again, I was supposed to go home, rest, and call with any changes. This time felt different. Crying out to God, I told him I was surrendered to His will. No matter what that meant, I wanted His will to unfold. Not mine.

I believe living in God's will is *the safest* place you can be. Bottom line: I trusted Him with everything, including our precious baby.

It was so hard to pray because in my mind and in my spirit, I knew what that meant, but my heart could not catch up. It was broken. Miscarrying a baby is one of the worst experiences I have ever lived through. The hours seemed like days and the days seemed like weeks. The physical pain pales in comparison to the helpless feeling of life slipping out of your body, one drop at a time. As a mommy, all you want to do is love and protect your babies.

Honestly, I think I cried until all the tears in my reservoirs were completely depleted.

After my appointment confirming our loss, I spoke with my mom about the hard stuff. All the things you think but you don't—or can't—say out loud. I had so many questions; my mind raced with all of the *why*s. But in those moments where I felt lost in tragedy, I felt God more. I felt His presence, love, and peace as He surrounded me. I realized I did not need to know the answers to my questions because God already did. I know our baby is in Heaven with Jesus, and one day we will be reunited. I have such a beautiful peace in knowing the first face she saw when she opened her eyes was His.

I have chosen to praise God continually and in all things. Through the good and through the heartache and tears, continually thanking Him for all He has done and continues to do in my life.

Our pastor says, "Worship is our warfare", and I believe that to be true because that's exactly what I continue to do and teach our babies to do. In the darkest storm, we worship and in the fiercest battles, we pray and call on the name of Jesus, so we can face every battle with faith and trust in Him. Even if it's just with the faith the size of a mustard seed.

Sisters, if you have lost a precious baby, I feel your pain. I cry out to God for you! I pray for you, even now, the same way I prayed that night on my knees in the shower. He is there with you at this very moment to comfort you, guide you, and give you a peace that transcends all knowledge.

He loves you in a way that no one else does or can. God's love is the only love that never fails or falters! First John 4:7–8 (NIV) says, "Dear friends, let us love one another, for love comes from God. Everyone who loves has been born of God and knows God. Whoever does not love does not know God, because GOD IS LOVE." Rest in that, Sisterhood. God's love is made complete in us.

My desire is that through this book, you will feel encouraged, inspired, and most of all, know you are not alone. No matter what you are facing, there is hope. "We can do all things through Christ who gives us strength." (Philippians 4:13, NLT) We are your Sisterhood, and we stand with you and your family. There are many times in life when I have felt like an old sweater, falling apart at the seams, and I needed God to sew me back together—again and again.

Each time, I have had to call on Him and ask Him for a healing hug. It is truly amazing every time I do this, for I can feel His presence and peace.

Dear Lord: Please reach down upon each person reading this book and give them a healing hug, increasing their faith exponentially and feeling your presence along the way.

Did you know the mustard seed is one of the tiniest seeds on Earth, yet grows into one of the largest garden plants? Our faith is comparable. It may be small at times, yet it is living and growing, if we allow it.

Remember Matthew 17:20 (NIV): *And He replied, "Because you have so little faith. Truly I tell you, if you have faith as small as a mustard seed, you can say to this mountain, 'Move from here to there,' and it will move. Nothing will be impossible for you."*

Let the journey begin. I am beyond blessed and honored to introduce you to some of the most courageous woman, those who were willing to share their journeys with the necklace.

These stories are authentic, powerful, and life changing. You must go on the journey with us, and I recommend grabbing a tissue or two.

First, I would like to introduce you to your "sister," Terrina.

2

Meet Terrina

New Faith, Big Hurts

My journey is filled with broken pieces, awful choices, and ugly truths. It's also filled with a major comeback, peace in my soul, and a grace that saved my life. One in eight women grieve from infertility. What is it about the infertility journey that is so messy and yet so beautiful at the same time? And where is God in the mist of it all? These were my questions and still are. Why did God choose me to be a one in eight?

Each of our stories takes on different appearances. Some of us can't walk through Target because, of course, they put the little girls' clothing at the front of the store.

We cry at the new Baby Gap commercials. We seem happy on the outside when we hear for the hundredth time that our neighbor is pregnant with her tenth kiddo. But secretly, our green jelly monster is sitting on our shoulders, haunting us, taunting, "Why her and not you?"

Some of us, we find temporary peace in the storm. We can seem so put together at times, but we are dying on the inside. We might even feel robbed. But if I were to speculate, go out on a limb, we all have been there or still are. Masks off, we are in this together—all of us. Infertility breaks us all into millions of shattered fragments . . . like the time when our patio table shattered into a pile of glass. The structure was still there—the frame survived—and from a distance, you could tell it was a table. But a useful table no more. We couldn't glue the glass back together. All we had left was the metal frame and air between the spaces. That's what infertility does to a woman. To a couple.

Infertility has brought so much shame and guilt to my home. Specifically, infertility has brought shame to me. "In his kindness God called you to share in his eternal glory by means of Christ Jesus. So after you have suffered a little while, he will restore, support, and strengthen you, and he will place you on a firm foundation." (1 Peter 5:10, NLT) I tell my story, not so I can get the glory, but so that others may know hope and find Jesus.

Unassuming Child

When I was six years old, my daddy dropped me off at kindergarten, in our small town. Maddox Elementary was one of five elementary schools that fed the local middle school. The kindergarten classroom was housed in the trailer building across from the main location. It was the summer of 1986.

Daddy came to pick me up just a few hours later, and my feet felt like they were incased with cement. My black-and-white saddle shoes so small, my toes had been trying to make a guest appearance all day. I desperately wanted to cut the tops off, so I could take some string I had found in my cubby and make my own sandals.

I felt shame for the first time that day. We didn't have the financial resources to get shoes that month. It never occurred to me that wearing blue jeans two inches too short and old GI Joe t-shirts was so I could hand them down to my younger brothers. I didn't own dresses, and I never had a doll to call my own.

Emotionally speaking, I don't know if there was a time I felt beautiful or heard the words, "I love you." Desperately wanting hair like Jessie Spano from *Saved by the Bell*—long, spiral, bouncy hair. She was beautiful. I wanted to be beautiful so that I could be loved. It was in the late '80s, and I was five years old raising my daddy and my two brothers.

My daddy had found himself at age twenty with a girl only fifteen-years-old and me. And by age twenty-four, two more babies had come along. My mother, the youngest of five, turned to sex and drugs for love. But that meant when there was no more sex, there was no more love. Soon after, she left, too.

My daddy, the boys, and I moved into Jessie Horn's two-bedroom home, my eighty-year-old great grandmother's home. She had an extra bedroom, and she offered to watch us at night so my daddy could work. Andrew, my youngest brother, was still small enough that he slept in a crib. Dusty, only fifteen months older, sometimes mistaken as Andrew's twin, slept in the dresser drawer, and my daddy laid his head on the floor at night. I had the privilege of sleeping in the only bed we owned. But it wasn't long before Dusty couldn't sleep in the old dresser we had purchased from Goodwill. It was time to move me into the same bedroom as my great grandmother, the one with the blue shag carpet. We shared bunk beds, which was fun for a five-year-old.

Grandma Jessie had been a devout Christian her whole life. Her husband had died when I was three years old. He was a good man. He was a great man! Grandma Jessie was a longtime member of the local Methodist church, located just blocks from her house, and every Sunday, she dragged us along. The church was enormous, and they made us run up and sit on the stage to sing, "Jesus Loves Us" before sending us back to the classrooms. "Who is this Jesus they talk about? I've never seen him," I thought to myself.

Daddy moved us from our GG's house two years later. I guess it was time for a new adventure. Little did I know, I wasn't going to see her much after that. Jessie died at the age of 101. Today, I know she is with our loving Father in Heaven. I'm not sure why she took on three babies, but she did. I'm not sure what her relationship was with Jesus, but I know that she loved and loved well. I bet she learned how from God, Himself. And after all, isn't that what Jesus commanded we all do?

"Give Me your Hand"

Times got tough. Daddy was on his second divorce by the time I was ten years old. Daddy and she were married only two long years. During the divorce, the ex-wife took all we had, including the refrigerator and our beds. No food, no bed, and soon no house. I can't say I blame her. She was an ordained minister at a church a few miles away. The holy Christians took up their stones and chucked them straight at her head. I believe they were intending to end her. They did that indeed, ended everyone in our house.

My father made a decision that day that God wasn't real any more, and we now had evidence. Daddy took a turn for the worse after she left, and he started drinking. The drinking was so bad; I learned to stay away for long periods of time. I snuck away in the middle of the night or didn't go home at all in hope someone would find me and take me away from the awful nightmare.

After a year, no one came to save me. As a young child, I had learned an overpowering message: this world is full of bad. And I'm bad. My dad doesn't want me, my mom didn't want me, and certainly, all that "unwanting" reinforced my strong belief that God didn't exist. At fifteen, I was looking for love in all the wrong places. Just like my mom. I became like the woman I didn't even know. I never wanted to be like my mother, but look at me. I wasn't any better than she was. I left home at sixteen years old and landed in any men's arms, anyone who would take me. I wish I could have just heard God tell me, "Give me your hand, My child."

At nineteen years old, I found myself sobbing on the bathroom toilet, holding news in my hands that pained me. I fell into complete denial, even as I stared between a pink "plus" and the man in my bed. My roommate came in and declared it was normal and not to panic. Every Tom, Dick, and Henry she knew had this happen to them. She had a way out for me. She reassured me that I was in no way meant to be a mom and couldn't be one. I quickly agreed. Once I kicked the tall stranger out of my apartment, we came up with a strategy to pay for it. I didn't have health insurance, and I was living paycheck to paycheck. I truly believed my choice wouldn't hurt anyone. I had convinced myself that was for the greater good.

I called my high school boyfriend and told him I needed him to help me.

Two things made Andy tick. One was sex and the other was money. First, I knew Andy couldn't afford another kid because he already had one when we were in high school. And second, Andy would help me pay my bills if I was short on money. I just had to pleasure him. I was a common-day Rahab.

Not Forgotten

Romans 8:1: "Therefore, there is now no condemnation for those who are in Christ Jesus."

Kelsey and I became colleagues in the fall of 2006, working for a local private school. She had a heavy-duty presence about her, a tough exterior and strong vocal opinions. Kelsey was my balance. Kelsey and I ran the same game. Party all night, repeat. We were likely covering up scars and battle wounds we both hid. Some, we had caused and some were inflicted by others. We just had to deal.

I couldn't tell by looking at her, and she didn't know it yet, but she had a great assignment from God, which she would have to carry out. Kelsey and I went our separate ways, but we always stayed in touch. To this day, as we live thousands of miles and an ocean apart, we are separated but never miss a beat when we do connect.

In 2008, the man who sat in front of me at the office and I became friends. A year later, we indulged in an office affair. He offered the love I was looking for. This time, he was more than a paycheck—more than just someone for pleasure. He and I connected. We married on the beaches of Jamaica. Little did I know that when we came back, many of my secrets would be exposed.

He had two boys, and they had lived bachelor lives for nearly four years before I came into the picture. Every Sunday, he and the boys would dress in their Sunday best and go to the same church where my "now husband" had grown up. I never joined them. The boys grew up there, too. It was a large church in the north part of town. A building made with red bricks, old linoleum tiles, and old-school ideas. Behind it sat an old farmhouse where the pastor lived.

My husband loved and lost greatly in his life. Between the loss of his father and his divorce from his first wife, my stance that God doesn't look out for anyone but Himself only strengthened. I doubted He even existed.

Rock Bottom

After nearly a year of trying to conceive, I grew tired. It was a job and a painful one at that. I couldn't stomach the idea of another negative pregnancy test. I stomped my way down the stairs and demanded we go to the doctor. My husband refused to acknowledge anything was wrong. I felt so broken. It brought back all the shame I had experienced when I was a child and throughout my adult life.

I knew why I couldn't have children. It's this crazy idea of karma. All the trouble I caused had led to this. It was coming back to bite me hard. Who was I kidding? My roommate from years ago was right all along. I wasn't mom material, and I started to believe I wasn't made to be a wife, either. The basic biological parts of me couldn't do what I tried to prevent all those years. I missed my only chance to be a mom. I tripped and fell into a dark hole, and I wasn't sure how I was going to get out of it. I didn't know how much my abortion had affected me until years later.

In the meantime, Kelsey, my colleague and friend from years ago, mentioned on Facebook she had started going to a local church, and she loved it. I was appalled. I couldn't believe she would betray me like that. I really needed someone to keep my misery company.

But I noticed small changes in her. She talked about how she was forgiven and this thing called grace was meeting her at the door. Still, I couldn't believe it. It had to be forged. Months passed by, my best friend found love, I didn't have a baby, and she was getting married. My own marriage was rocky. The building blocks had been knocked down, smashed and burned. I needed something bigger than me. For the first time in my life, I couldn't manipulate, control, or ignore my story. I knew I had to rebuild, but I didn't know where to start. I hit rock bottom.

Kelsey would be the first one to introduce me to Jesus. I was knee-deep in my own disease, and I needed relief. I called her one night and asked if I could go to church with her. She was stunned, but I took her answer as a "yes."

Walking into the church auditorium that morning and sitting in the chair, I started to feel as if I had made a mistake by coming. I wanted this day to be different. I couldn't keep living in this garbage. I swallowed my doubts and sat down with a huge sigh. Sweat wet my palms, and my heart raced. Faces I didn't know introduced themselves to me with big smiles. Kelsey looked over and gave me a wink. I slowly counted to five and thought, "I don't have to be brave, just have a little courage."

It was irrational, but I thought, "I might get stoned by all the Christians," just like my daddy's ex-wife had been twenty years before. The pastor stood on stage and gave his message. I couldn't tell you what it was about, but after he was done, in a short twenty minutes, I heard him say, "God, I believe someone came here today needing to hear from You." I closed my eyes and thought, "How in the world did he know?" Fear erupted. I closed my eyes and chitchatted with God for a minute. Tears streamed down my face as I asked Him for His help. I told Him I didn't deserve it, but if He would let me and Help me, I would forever be His child. In that moment, I changed my mind about God, which then forever changed my life.

Anthony

I was getting ready for work one morning when I heard a voice on the morning news. They were highlighting one of the kiddos in foster care who was looking for a "forever family." I'll never forget that little boy's voice. As I peered at the TV, I saw a familiar face. Anthony was now a young Black man. I knew him when he was only eight years old, and I never saw him again after the authorities took him from his grandma. Thirteen now, his smile had never changed. My heart sang, and I thought, "This is God telling me I am going to be his mom." My husband and I jumped right into the process.

We began our foster care courses with the intention that we would adopt Anthony. Three months into the process, I received a phone call I didn't expect. Anthony was not going to be ours. I was heart broken. I couldn't comprehend why God would put this guy back in my life again but not let me have him. Chances were he wasn't going to be with any family but remain in the system. "I will not leave you as orphans; I am coming to you." (John 14:18, CSB) I hang onto that for him. I pray that one day, he will know this kind of love.

In next to no time, I was learning how to live in the dark. As I read the Bible, I learned that God teaches His children to live by faith and not by sight. That's why we have to go through darkness. He has to take light away so we can't always see. No one told me it would be easy, but I'm not sure I was prepared for how hard the next five years would turn out to be. The God I just met wanted to use me, but I wasn't sure for what. When I found out Anthony wasn't going to be our son, I was left questioning God, asking Him why He put Anthony on the news and then didn't allow him to come home? Over the next few years, I leaned into bad theology. The idea I lived was if I worked harder and harder, God would accept me, and He would reward me with a family.

In December 2011, I went to my doctor for medical advice. One month later, January 2012, they found twenty-eight fibroid tumors on my uterus. Without the removal of these masses, I would never have children. And if I have them removed, my odds were almost as high that I wouldn't have kids because of the damage it could cause.

Mustard Seeds

Standing in my kitchen, I prepared a meal for my friends who were coming over that evening. Niki and her mother were a part of that group. Niki was *that person* everyone wanted to do life with. Her kindness was infectious. She truly lived her life as a "Proverbs 31 woman." She was beautiful on the outside, but I always thought it was because her beauty came from inside. And she must have learned it from her mom. Momma, as we lovingly referred to her, treated us with respect and love. She always had an open home but was never afraid to tell it to you like a mom when you needed a stern hand. Niki and her mother, Momma, held out a card for me as a gift. Inside was a keychain holding a tiny mustard seed, one similar to the seed Niki wore in a necklace as she tried to conceive her first baby.

Symbolic of Matthew 17:20 (NIV), *He replied, "Because you have so little faith. Truly I tell you, if you have faith as small as a mustard seed, you can say to this mountain, 'Move from here to there,' and it will move. Nothing will be impossible for you."*

I carried the mustard seed to remind me to keep my faith until one Sunday morning at church. While Niki and I acted as greeters at the door during worship, she asked if she could share something else with me. She took her mustard seed necklace off and gave it to me. We prayed over it and put it around my neck. She wore it while she went through her journey and now it was mine to wear on my journey. On the outside of the necklace was written, "All Things Are Possible." I would wear that necklace for the next three and a half years.

I wore the necklace, not as a good luck charm, but more as a reminder. The night she gave me the necklace, I decided to remove my tumors. My surgery lasted five hours. My recovery was excruciating and slow-going. Still, we didn't know if I was going to be able to have kids. But all I needed was a little bit of faith. Just the amount equal to the size of a mustard seed.

My first IUI (intrauterine insemination) was scheduled, and I couldn't have been more excited. I grew two eggs, and it was a textbook process until the morning of the procedure. But I had faith.

It was not successful. I was upset but still grabbed hold of my faith, telling myself it would work. Round two came and went. Not successful again. The third time, what I had hoped would be the last, was not successful, either. It was awful. I was trying to not go back to my old thoughts, to lose my faith, but by this time, I couldn't help myself. I had failed God over and over, and I was being punished for all the years I had offended Him. I agonized daily.

Long-Term Visitors

Leo and Heaven came to live with us after our third attempt of IUI. I believe God was asking me to watch over His children even in the mist of my pain. So I did. During their stay with us we received two different calls from two different originations—a local county attorney and a personal friend. Both had opportunities for us to grow our family. At the same time, they both fell apart. I started to feel God might have abandoned me. Leo and Heaven left our home, and we found our bank account basically at zero. There was no way we could continue fertility treatments. We needed a miracle, and I needed hope.

The Bible taught me something during this time in my life. There was a man in the Book of Genesis named Jacob. Jacob was one of two sons of Isaac and Rebekah. Esau was a man's man. And Jacob was quiet and cared for the flocks. Jacob had some issues. As the story goes, Jacob wrestles with God all night. As he wrestled, God's presence became more and more real to him. And the fact that it lasted all night is significant. The darkness symbolized Jacob's situation, and it symbolized mine. When I was ready to hold on, the Lord was there, ready to help me. I knew I needed to tell someone about my past so I could move on with my future. I was ready and I knew who that somebody would be.

It wasn't that I didn't trust my husband, but I felt that our marriage had a lot of stress on it as it was. I needed someone to extend grace. I needed someone who loved me and still would after my dark secrets were revealed. It was easy to decide that it would be Niki and Momma. I told them how I felt God was punishing, me and I shared about all the shame I carried. I had chosen an abortion in my past, and I couldn't forgive myself. I had slept around. I couldn't forgive myself for that either. I couldn't get pregnant, and I couldn't forgive myself. I had been practicing bad theology—that I had to do more to be given a second chance. I didn't want to go to Heaven and have God say, "Well, you are going to miss out because you didn't do everything I asked." Or, "I don't allow your kind here." I needed to extend grace to myself. I couldn't pretend to be someone I wasn't. I was broken. Niki and her mom held my hand as the streams of tears fell to the floor. Momma reminded me that God doesn't work like that. I was made new the day I decided to let Jesus into my heart. I was forgiven. Nothing could take that from me. Her tenderness was the salve I needed to start healing.

It costs roughly $1,200 for each IUI attempt. It costs $1,400 a month to raise two kids in the system for nine months. But just like Jesus, that was Friday. On Sunday, God blessed me. It was as if He finally heard me let go of all my anger, regret, and sorrow. He had been catching every tear for thirty-four years. And now, it was His time.

I was going through a stack of checks that had been donated to my husband and me once our story was made public. I was speechless. I couldn't have asked for a better gift. No matter the size of the donation, each one from this group of people came through for us. They believed in us. I suppose people saw their reflections in us. I didn't feel dirty any longer. When I got to the bottom of the pile, there was an anonymous, certified check for twenty thousand dollars. *What!* Could it really be? No one does this! I could only explain it as God giving me a new name. I was His child and He had heard my cries.

It was a new start. I put my head on straight and would try not to look back any longer. I will always walk with a thorn in my side. Just as Paul pleaded with God three times, I would plead multiples of that number. But God's grace was enough for the Apostle Paul, and "His power was made perfect in Paul's weakness." (2 Cor. 12:9) Hash tag, "same here."

It was IUI day, again! And once again, it failed. On attempt number seven, we were finally pregnant! I found out on my birthday, and at my party, I couldn't help but let everyone know. What better gift could I have gotten? It was better than anything I could have dreamed. On Monday, at work during a meeting, I had a horrible feeling something was wrong. I went to the bathroom, and there I saw I had lost my baby. It was the most sobering feeling I'd ever had. That day, I went home and sat on my bathroom floor and wept. I prayed for hours. That day felt like it went on for hundreds of hours. I was exhausted. I needed time to heal. Jesus learned obedience from suffering. I had felt a measure of that weight.

It will always bring me great joy to picture the day I will get to meet my beautiful babies in Heaven. I rejoice in the fact that Jesus was there to take them by the hand and hold them until I am reunited with them once again.

The Book of Matthew

Jordan, a very sweet young woman, approached me one morning. She had a puzzled look on her face. Almost as puzzling as what was about to come out of her mouth. "This is going to seem weird," she said, "but God told me He wants you to fast and read the Book of Matthew."

The same day, a man named Dean came over to deliver a message to me: "God told me to tell you He hasn't forgotten you." *I couldn't dream this up, even if I tried.* Every day, leading up to these encounters, I had imagined Jesus sitting next to me in my two-hour commute to the office. He would just sit and listen. I would sing Him a song if I had nothing to say. But mostly, I would converse about my feelings and how I knew He loved me. That the disappointments I felt were only temporary, but I needed Him to help me through them. Jeremiah 29:11 says, "For I know the plan I have for you,' declares the Lord, 'plans to prospers you and not to harm you, plans to give you hope and a future."

The Bible gives us four accounts of Jesus' life, referred to as The Gospels. Each of these books covers a lot of the same topics but from the different perspectives of the different authors. There are Mark, Luke, Matthew, and John. The Book of Matthew was written anonymously but believed to have been written by Matthew, one of the twelve apostles. In the beginning, we see that Matthew includes some women's genealogy. These women were Tamar, Rahab, Ruth, Bathsheba, and Mary. Of course, God wanted me to read this book. Tamar pretended to be a prostitute, Rahab was a prostitute, Ruth married into a land that was forbidden, Bathsheba committed adultery with David, and Mary . . . she was an unmarried teenager. Of course, God wanted me to read this book! He was preparing me for my God Story of redemption. I learned a lot from this author.

IVF

One afternoon, my husband went to a company event and ran into the operations managers at a fertility clinic. He told our story and the man extended an offer to help. We met with the doctor and decided to start our IVF (in-vitro fertilization) journey shortly after. We had half of the donated money left, but IVF is an expensive option. We opened four new credit cards, the nurse collected donated medication, and we began. Things seemed promising. Then, I received a phone call from my nurse. Another surgery was in my future. My tumors were back. I went home and prayed. Christianity has never been easy for me. But I had experienced great pain before, so I held strong to God's promises. He would never leave me nor forsake me.

On the way to the operating room, my surgeon suddenly turned around and got down on his knee. My heart fluttered. *What is he doing?*

"I changed my mind." *What? You can't change your mind now.*

He explained he would only do the bare minimum, and I'd be home in no time. He said he had a "Jesus moment" and wanted to give me the best opportunities he could.

Transfer Day

The night before the embryo transfer, I was working at a client's site when I received a call. I was not expecting anything out of the ordinary, but an unknown spot had appeared on my last ultrasound. No, I wouldn't accept it. I claimed it in Jesus' name! "Because of your faith, it will happen." (Matthew 9:29, NIV)

I stood up from my desk in astonishment. The transfer was going to be cancelled. My jaw dropped. I prayed in my car; I prayed in my bedroom, and that morning, I still believed the medical team would change its verdict. God says to "cast my cares on him," so I did. Casting cares before I even understood what anxiety was. I've been a worrier my entire life. I can't make a decision if I don't first sleep on it and pass it through at least a dozen scenarios. Naturally, I had a Plan *B* for everything, including what I would do if I got on a plane and it was crashing. But this situation wasn't changing, and I couldn't implement any Plan *B*s.

In fact, the same image showed up on the second attempt of FET transfer. But once again, I stood with God. "Be still and know I am God." (Psalm 46:10)

This verse—"Be still"—wasn't what I thought it was. It doesn't ask us to stop doing what we're doing but to shut down our worries and our own planning efforts. That's what I did. They had no room in my house any longer. "Hey, Devil! I'm not going to give you any more time, attention, or energy. You have no place here!" That day, I made a sign and hung it in my house.

God makes mountains move. The image that appeared on my ultrasound the first and second time disappeared in the morning. I had, for the first time, learned to live in the darkness, and now, I could stand and say I saw it through.

I was going to get to transfer my babies. Leading up to this excitement, I had a very candid conversation with my doctor. He explained that I didn't have much more than a twenty-five percent chance of conceiving. Truthfully, Doctor Riggs mentioned we might want to look at surrogacy. But I looked at my sign and said, "No more fear." I am not going to live in fear any longer. I punched that idea square in its mock turtleneck. *Let's do this.*

Ten days later, I was teaching a class when the phone rang, and I stepped away to take it. That conversation, although brief, will forever play in my head. "Terrina, we need you to come in tomorrow. You are pregnant."

James 1:2–4: "Consider it pure joy, my brothers and sisters, whenever you face trials of many kinds, because you know that the testing of your faith produces perseverance. Let perseverance finish its work so that you may be mature and complete, not lacking anything." I was going to be a mom!

It was a hurry-up-and-wait process. But when it was done, everything slammed right into place. If the truth is told, I was terrified. With normal pregnancies, mothers can be nervous. Some mothers go through forty weeks of pure bliss and some mothers never get to take their babies home. Most others fall in the middle somewhere. My heart goes out to all of you. Mommies are given a monumental task, and although we do everything we can, there will be fellow mommies amongst us who will have to say good-bye too early.

My feelings were magnified a hundred times over. At twenty-two weeks, I went into labor. The doctors were able to stop it, but I was forced to reside inside my bedroom for nearly eleven weeks to hang on as long as I could.

On My Way to Heaven

Exactly thirty-three weeks into my pregnancy I had conversations with my doctors that I would soon be delivering. I prepped to have a C-section.

"I had a feeling that this was going to happen." We've all said that at some point. For me, intuition was heightened by the Holy Spirit. That day, I knew something was off; something was terribly wrong. I was wheeled into the operating room, and within ten minutes, my first baby, Tennyson Faith, was born. I heard her cry, the most magnificent sound to ever hit my ears. Tilly Grace was delivered two minutes later. I couldn't breathe. My eyes drew shut and my head was hitting the steel table. It was a real-life emergency made for movies. The nurses rushed my husband and my newborn baby girls out of the room. I lay dying.

I had placenta increta, which had gone undiagnosed. I looked up at the man above my head and whispered to him, "I am dying, and I want to tell my husband goodbye." I assumed I was leaving my husband to raise two beautiful baby girls.

I had two blood transfusions, totaling seventeen units of blood. And after nine hours in the operating room, I woke up in the ICU, thirty hours later. Most mommies don't survive, but God allowed me more days to live here on Earth.

Why was I chosen to be one in eight? I'll tell you what I know. I don't understand the whole picture yet, but I get to see glimpses of my children and the impact they will make on this world. I am able to deliver flowers to someone's doorstep when they get the disappointing news that only one embryo survived after they spent thirty thousand dollars to have a baby. I'd be here to hold a fellow mom in my arms in a hospital bed while her baby lays next to her, breathless, because he didn't make it. I will pick up the homeless mother to take her to the hospital to deliver her health baby boy. I will pick up a child from the doorstep of Social Services just to give them a drink. I will celebrate overcoming addiction, recovery, and The Gospel every day.

These weren't my plans for my life, but God has greater plans for all of us. Better than we can ever imagine.

God does things in our darkness, in our storms, and in the midst of our pain. God put stars in the sky so we can know He is there. Our stories don't always end the way we want, but sometimes, they end better. In spite of everything you and I have done, Jesus thought we were worth dying for.

Dear God, there are so many of us in the middle of a journey that we don't understand. We feel that we don't deserve or don't see a way out. You are a good, good Father. As our good, good Father, You provide us with all the necessities, and You hear our cries. You believe in us and love us as You only want life abundantly for us. Father, as we navigate our lives, we have made mistakes and carry those hurts with us. Please forgive us as we recognize that hurt doesn't help us. Your Son Jesus has already taken care of all that, and all You need us to do is to believe You are still with us. I pray that this book, this comeback of mine, this story, gives women all over the world new hope. I pray my children know how much they are loved, even before I held them in my arms. I pray they know the two people who would die for them, Jesus and me. I pray that the husbands who watch their wives go through this pain know how much God loves them, too. I pray that the mommies who've had to say good-bye to their babies know how close You are to them. I pray the mommies who are barren will have this mi-

raculous encounter with You and You will light their paths, as You did mine. Please bring strong women into their lives to hold their arms up when they don't have the strength to move forward. God, I know You have amazing plans for each and every one here on Earth. I pray that every mother, daughter, and child grows to know You and understands just how much You love them, amen.

Tennyson Faith and Tilly Grace will forever remind me as long as they walk this earth that God will break down any wall, climb any mountain, and light up any darkness in my life to find me. He will leave the ninety-nine for me.

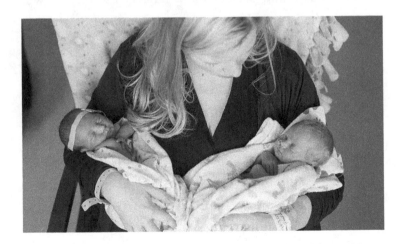

****

Amen, Terrina . . . Amen!

Sisterhood, I imagine you are wiping your eyes and feeling a range of emotions sweeping through your body after reading sweet T's story, just as I did. Emotions may be ranging from compassion to inspiration!

Don't worry; I will give her an extra hug and a high-five for you!

The three T's! Terrina, Tenny, and Tilly! They are indeed an inspiration and living proof that with God, all things are possible. God's grace is fresh and new every day, and it is for each of us! 2 Corinthians 12:8–9 (NIV) says, "Three times I pleaded with the Lord to take it away from me. But he said to me, 'My grace is sufficient for you, for my power is made perfect in weakness. Therefore I will boast all the more gladly about my weaknesses, so that Christ's power may rest on me.'"

Terrina's vulnerability and transparency is absolutely beautiful and speaks volumes about her character. One full of strength, kindness, truth and love! In times of darkness, she always finds her way to the light and manages to let it shine bright. Every time I hear the song, "This Little Light of Mine," I think of our sweet T!

She is a true "Proverbs 31 Woman" with a heart of gold! A beautiful soul and dear friend!

She and her husband, Dean, never give up; they always hope and believe for the best, no matter what and thankfully, they are living their happily ever after!

As you reflect on Terrina's incredible story, remember, no matter how dark it may seem, there is always light at the end of the tunnel. Sometimes, our answers don't come overnight. Sometimes, they take weeks, months, or even years. But take heart and grab a hold of your faith, just as T did. Your journey is exactly that—your beautiful journey. It is not a destination; it is a spiritual and physical trek unique to you and your family; stay strong and hopeful, and know that we are here to support you. The Sisterhood continues.

Terrina passed her necklace to our dear, sweet, beautiful friend, Stephanie.

Stephanie holds a special place in our hearts. Although she is younger in numerical age, her soul is wise beyond her years.

It is my pleasure to introduce you to your "sister," Stephanie.

3

Meet Stephanie

Love Never Ends

Someone could drop a baby off on my front door step right now, and I would have absolutely everything needed to take care of that little one: a nursery, the tiny, adorable outfits, stacks of diapers, and an open heart. It is with both hope and heartbreak that I have gotten to this place.

Ever since my husband and I started talking about the hope that we had for our future children, everything became about Beau. We knew that's what we wanted to name our son, and every thought we had about children included a dream of what Beau's life with us would be like.

We tried immediately for him. By immediately, I mean on our wedding night. Because that's how badly we wanted to be parents, even though it was sort of insane. So, of course, I was pretty heartbroken when we weren't magically pregnant after one week of trying. And the painful strings to our hearts kept coming undone when we found out other family members were getting pregnant before us. The mommas-to-be would tell me, "Oh, it will happen soon for you, and then we will be sharing this magical experience together!"

Then those babies were born. And soon grew out of their newborn outfits. And took their first steps. And I was still empty-armed.

I had started to feel there might be something wrong very early into our trying. We hadn't been actually "trying" that long, but we certainly hadn't been preventing for quite a while. So I decided to get everything checked out. Just to be sure it really was all just in my head. Or that all I had to do was "just relax," as every person tells you when you're experiencing infertility.

At the same time I began fertility tests, my mother was diagnosed with end-stage breast cancer. My mother suffered from deep depression, and she had been hiding her breast cancer for years—until it became unbearable. Her cancer was so advanced that she had to quit working and move in with my husband and me right away. Admittedly, I was sort of excited to have her move in with us, at first, because I wanted to rescue her. She had been independent for so long that I felt like she just needed to breathe a little and let me take care of her. One month after she moved in with us, I had my first uterine test for infertility.

My doctor explained that during the uterine test, I should feel some pressure. But something he failed to tell me (and probably for a good reason, if I'm being honest) is that pressure feels a lot like pain, and it's very hard for your brain to distinguish between the two. I screamed on that table. Thank goodness it only lasted thirty seconds. I sat up, and was forced to take deep breaths for what felt like forever before I could walk out of there. I met the doctor back in his office where he diagnosed me with severe endometriosis, which was forcing my fallopian tubes closed. He had a pretty positive and upbeat attitude about it, telling me this wasn't a deal breaker; so I wasn't totally heartbroken as I left that appointment. Just shaking with anxiety.

A few weeks later, I still hadn't gotten my period. At first, I thought the test, which had forced fluid through my tubes had just screwed everything up. Then, I started to question if I was pregnant. I made myself wait until I was one week late to take a test.

It was a Tuesday morning when I woke up at 5:00 a.m. and sprang out of bed to take that test. I had taken countless tests before, so my expectations were low; I harbored a negative thought process in general about pregnancy tests. But this time felt different. I felt positive . .

. and it was positive. The uterine test had opened up my fallopian tubes just enough to make this work. So the pain was worth it!

I launched into bed to tell my sleepy husband that we were officially expecting. He lit up instantly and kissed my belly and whispered, "Beau."

That Friday, I sat in the parking lot of a pharmacy, waiting on my mother to pick up her new prescriptions. I felt something "down there" that didn't seem right for a pregnancy. I drove us home, trying not to show the fear that was taking over.

My doctor told me she needed to see me right away, to determine if I was miscarrying. I ran downstairs, trembling. When my mother asked me what was wrong, I couldn't hold back anymore. I told her that I might be having a miscarriage. She came with me to the doctor's appointment. They couldn't find a heartbeat, but I was also so early in my pregnancy that there might not even be one yet. So I was scheduled to return on Monday for another blood test and then, we would know. We got home from the appointment, and my mom lit up. "I'm going to be a grandma!" I knew I shouldn't let her get too excited, but it was rare to see a smile spreading across her face. I couldn't crush her delight.

That weekend was Father's Day Weekend. That weekend was spent treating myself like glass. I thought sitting down incorrectly would shatter the baby inside me. Our parents, meanwhile, were telling my husband, "Happy Father's Day!"

Monday came. So did the confirmation of my miscarriage. I broke down on the kitchen floor with my mother. I was so angry with God. Knowing other people get to be parents, even when they mistreated and ignored their other children, tore me to shreds. It's one of the thought patterns I have struggled with most in my journey to parenthood. *Why does God allow people who don't even want children, or don't treat their current children kindly, to have children?* Obviously, I still don't know the answer.

Weeks later, I took my mom to church one day. My friends from church lit up when I showed up with my mom and said they had something for me. They both came up to me and put their hands on my shoulders while I opened their gift. Tears erupted. I knew it was something to bring me hope. I hadn't even gotten that little box opened yet, but I knew it.

Inside the box was a necklace with a round charm with a mustard seed in the middle. Around the mustard seed were the words, "All things are possible." This gift from two friends who had both walked their own unique journeys through infertility spoke volumes. As they told me the story of Jesus and the disciples and the mustard seed, I continued to sob while stroking the little pendant with my fingers.

I wore that necklace every day. I wore it through continued fertility tests. Through IUI treatments. Through the pregnancies and births of friends' babies. And through the death of my mother.

My brother called me out of the blue one night when our mother had really started to take a downward path. My husband and I had sold our home two months prior to pay for IVF, forcing my mother to live in an apartment with my brother while I lived with my in-laws. It had been a difficult decision.

"I just can't take care of her anymore. I don't know what to do. We have to take her to the hospital, so they can try to get her into a care facility," he said.

I considered waiting until the morning to go get her, but at the urging of my mother-in-law, my husband, and a friend of ours, I drove to my brother's apartment to get her. She was cold and pale when we arrived. The guys carried her down the stairs.

She was unconscious in the hospital for several days. She only had a few stable days in the hospital when she made any sense, but she had a breathing tube in.

One day, she was lying in bed awake, so I told her what I had been up to that day. I mentioned something related to the fertility treatments we had just been through. We had done our first egg retrieval, which started off beautifully but quickly went downhill. Thirteen embryos decreased to one embryo, which then became one unhealthy embryo. Back to square one.

Whatever I said to my mother about the treatments that day, she responded with a clear message: "Don't wait." Despite the breathing tube, she spoke to me. I knew what she meant. She didn't want her death to become a reason why I would wait to become a mother. I knew she had comfort in going Home, that she would hold my lost baby in her arms for me, until I arrived.

I kept going strong after she passed away, continuing with my new vitamin and acupuncture regimen, set by my new doctor. A few months later, we were ready for a new round of IVF. They did things differently this time, and I did, too. We retrieved more eggs. I kept telling myself, "Have faith."

Twenty-six eggs became eight embryos, which dwindled down to one embryo. I crashed into the negativity though patterns of old when I was asked if I wanted to send this embryo to testing to make sure it was healthy. At the clinic we used, you could only transfer healthy embryos. So to not test the embryo was to give it no chance. The only reason I sent it for testing was because it was free, part of what we had already paid.

I counted that embryo down and out. I had already moved my thinking and planning heart onto the next steps. "What will we do now that IVF has failed us twice?"

I was home one day, battling a severe case of vertigo (in general, I think my body dislikes me), while my mother-in-law was downstairs, having an employee meeting. My phone rang.

After I hung up, I clumsily sprinted downstairs and screamed to my mother-in-law, "I have a healthy embryo!" We jumped and cried and screamed with excitement. When she asked me about the gender, I realized I had completely forgotten to ask the nurse. When my transfer nurse called me a few weeks later, I caved and asked her for the gender. Boy. *Beau.*

The news of our soon-to-be pregnancy was the most exciting thing in the world for us. It was all I could think about. My whole life became focused on getting ready for this little boy. I painted the nursery before my transfer. My husband, who houses some of the same negativity I do, asked, "What happens if this doesn't work? Then, we'll have to look at this empty, painted room all the time. We'll have to just shut the door." I decided to have faith instead.

After my embryo transfer, I took two full weeks off from work, despite the nurses telling me only a few days was necessary. I wanted to give Beau every chance I could. I lay around on the couch for two weeks, watching every horrendous movie I could to keep my mind off wondering if the transfer had worked.

The day of my pregnancy blood test might be one of the longest days in my human existence. I forced myself to put my phone down and walk away. But not too far away, of course. I was expecting that all-important phone call. The tone in my nurse's voice said it all when I answered my phone. Our pregnancy test was positive.

This time felt different. I knew for a fact that Beau was a healthy embryo; I had a team of highly trained embryologists who had confirmed that. So miscarrying him due to my egg health wasn't a concern. I treated myself like a fragile flower during my first trimester, just to be extra careful. Still having faith but realizing it was a delicate situation.

The majority of my pregnancy felt like I was constantly holding my breath. I reached the five weeks and three days mark—the point at which I had miscarried our first baby. I got to twelve weeks—the point at which my sister-in-law had miscarried her third baby. I got to twenty weeks—the point at which my friend had miscarried her twins. I got to twenty-six weeks—the point at which my friend had lost her baby to preeclampsia.

At twenty weeks, I had been diagnosed with complete placenta previa, meaning that my placenta was covering my cervix; and therefore, I could not have a typical delivery. I was okay with not delivering "normally" and having to do a C-section instead. But I was worried about the other complications, ones that meant I could lose my baby.

At my thirty-two-week check-up, I was expecting to hear that my placenta hadn't moved and that we would be scheduling my C-section for five weeks later. So, of course,

I had a five-minute panic attack when I was told that it had moved, and I would, in fact, be planning to deliver normally. I wasn't prepared for the thought of actually having to push a baby out, and eight weeks wasn't enough time to wrap my head around that!

But I prepared nonetheless. We took our breastfeeding class and our birth class. And we inched closer to the end of my pregnancy. I started having false contractions just shy of week thirty-eight. So they wouldn't induce me. By the time I hit thirty-eight weeks a few days later, they had stopped. I spent the last two weeks of my pregnancy barely sleeping, lying awake on the couch at night in excitement and delirium that soon, Beau would be here.

At forty weeks and two days, my husband stayed up late, not heading to bed until midnight. I was asleep for several hours, but I needed to get up to go to the bathroom and then went back to bed. As I sat down on the bed, I felt a warm gush of fluid. I looked down with unease, expecting to see blood. I don't know why, but in my heart, I assumed it would be blood. And it was. I was so shaken that I told my husband to call the doctor. At midnight, that meant waiting up to an hour to hear back from the on-call doctor. Luckily, my husband was thinking more clearly than I was and yelled to his parents to call an ambulance. I went to the bathroom to clean up and change my clothes. Then, I calmly sat on the stairs, waiting for the ambulance, while the rest of the house was engulfed in chaos.

When the paramedics got there, they put me on a stretcher and took me outside. One of them ran up to our bedroom to see exactly how much blood there was. They quickly decided to take me to the nearest hospital instead of the one I was scheduled to deliver at, the one where my doctor had privileges. Instead, they took me to the hospital where my mother died.

Those early hours of that morning are a blur. I arrived at the hospital to a team of nurses who thought I still had placenta previa, but I corrected them, explaining I no longer had it. Then, I went upstairs and was in so much pain already from contractions that they gave me an epidural right away. The doctor ordered an ultrasound, so I waited. Later that morning, they finally came and did my ultrasound, confirming that Beau was okay. I had a partial placental abruption, but as far as they could tell, I was okay to deliver. They induced me. They measured Beau at eight pounds, eleven ounces, which was a lot bigger than the last measurement my doctors had done.

We laid around all day in the hospital in excitement. Everyone ate quietly around me, for I was not even allowed to think about eating, let alone take a drink of water. One of my closest friends brought me a Sprite to drink immediately after delivery because it was all I could think about.

Around 5:00 p.m., I was dilated enough to begin pushing. My husband and I, having just spent all but eight months of our marriage living with parents, decided we wanted to be in the room alone. So everyone left for the waiting room.

Within the first hour, we knew Beau was turned sideways and needed to be shifted. We tried everything to get him to turn. Shift change came, and we got a new nurse and a new on-call doctor. Over the next few hours, we tried every method they suggested to get him out. I had been pushing for four hours when my husband asked, "When are we just going to call it?" My doctor assured me that I wasn't pushing hard enough and wasn't pushing correctly, and that if I could, he would be there in twenty minutes. Despite my crying and pleading that I just didn't have it in me, I kept on pushing.

At 11:00 p.m., six hours into pushing, my doctor made me take a nap. She thought I was too tired to push correctly. So I napped for what everyone later told me was forty-five minutes (and not seconds as it felt to me), and then I was woken up to keep pushing. We tried for a short while longer before my doctor called it. She was taking me in for a C-section. We were so relieved. He would be here soon, and this nightmare would be over.

In the hallway on the way to the OR, they lost his heartbeat. My C-section became an emergency. And the pressure of them cutting into me felt a lot like pain. Yet again, I was screaming on a table waiting for something to be over. I heard the anesthesiologist say, "Baby!" when the pressure finally stopped. I was exhausted. I tried to get out the words to ask why Beau wasn't crying, but I couldn't form them. Instead, I passed out.

When I woke up, my first sight was a nurse crying uncontrollably. I didn't understand why she was crying. She stepped to the side, and I saw my husband holding a bundle of blankets, crying in a way I had only seen him cry several times before. Someone behind me finally said, "I'm sorry, but we lost the baby." I started crying out, "No!" It was the only word I could form before I passed out again.

I finally woke up in a new room with my husband beside me, holding the same bundle of blankets. He asked me if I wanted to hold him. I declined. I thought, "What am I thinking? This is my little boy. I want him next to me." I could barely move, but I snuggled him next to me while I sobbed.

The forty weeks that I had with Beau were enough for me to love him through this lifetime and the next. He was born and died at 12:35 a.m. on October 9th. I have a large clock in our kitchen stopped at 12:35 because that is the time that our lives stood still . . . forever. Every thought I have of Beau, I picture his tiny, perfectly round face. I know everyone says their baby is the prettiest baby ever, but I *know* that Beau truly was. He was too perfect for this earth.

I take small bits of comfort knowing that Beau is with my mom, being held by her for me until the moment I can scoop him up in my arms and hold him in the way that my arms have been aching to do ever since we lost him.

Losing a child requires an immense amount of faith. An amount that I'm not sure I possess. But I know that if I have faith the size of a mustard seed, every mountain that stands in front of me can be moved. I have moved a mountain of grief, and even though it still exists, and I have to visit it from time to time, it doesn't need to stand in my way of seeing a brighter future.

We have faith that a future exists for us, one where a child on this earth, who was born to someone else, will need us, and we will be chosen to raise that child with the same love and hope that we feel in our hearts for Beau. And we can tell that child all about their big brother in Heaven who is waiting for all of us with an open heart.

I wear my necklace each day as my heart prepares for this next adventure. One that will require an immeasurable amount of faith, I'm sure.

****

Weeping best describes my reaction to reading Stephanie's story, one written in her own powerful words, and I know God weeps with us.

Psalm 56:8 (NLT) reads, "You keep track of all my sorrows. You have collected all my tears in your bottle. You have recorded each one in your book."

In times of our deepest sorrow God is with us and He cares about every detail of our lives and every tear we shed. His love for us is infinite; it is a love that never fails and never ends.

In the years I have known Stephanie, she has been through more than most should experience in a lifetime. The grief she has endured is unimaginable, but if you look into her eyes, all you see is love.

1 Corinthians 13:

If I speak in the tongues of men and of angels, but have not love, I am a noisy gong or a clanging cymbal. And if I have prophetic powers, and understand all mysteries and all knowledge, and if I have all faith, so as to remove mountains, but have not love, I am nothing. If I give away all I have, and if I deliver up my body to be burned, but have not love, I gain nothing.

Love is patient and kind; love does not envy or boast; it is not arrogant or rude. It does not insist on its own way; it is not irritable or resentful; it does not rejoice at wrongdoing, but rejoices with the truth. Love bears all things, believes all things, hopes all things, endures all things.

Love never ends. As for prophecies, they will pass away; as for tongues, they will cease; as for knowledge, it will pass away. For we know in part and we prophesy in part, but when the perfect comes, the partial will pass away. When I was a child, I spoke like a child, I thought like a child, I reasoned like a child. When I became a man, I gave up childish ways. For now we see in a mirror dimly, but then face to face. Now I know in part; then I shall know fully, even as I have been fully known.

So now faith, hope, and love abide, these three; but the greatest of these is love.

Stephanie exudes love in the way she lives her life and cares for others. Although most would get lost in the grief she has experienced, she remains hopeful and stands in faith for her future. She is a woman of strength and courage and knows that God has big plans for their family. Members of the Sisterhood stand in faith with us while Stephanie and Tyler's journey continues. What a joy it will be to watch their family grow!

Update: SISTERS! [Picture me on a megaphone . . . now, start the drumroll please!]

I am so happy and honored to share with you that Stephanie and Tyler have welcomed their beautiful and perfect son, Hudson, into the world!

This picture is priceless!

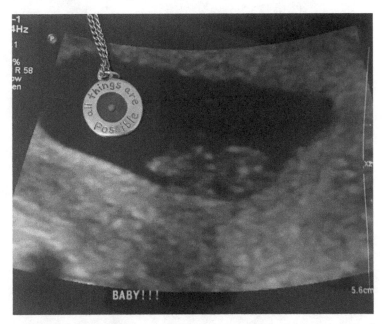

Stephanie, I am proud of you and love you beyond measure. I know your mom is delighted in the way you live your life with such passion and bravery, just as she did.

We honor and remember your cherished son, Beau, and beautiful mother, Marcy. We know they are with Jesus, and we stand in hope, knowing we will see them again and that you will have the desire of your heart to hold Beau in your loving arms again.

As most great stories do, the story of the necklace had already taken on a life of its own. You see, before Beau was born, Stephanie passed her necklace on to someone close to her that needed it on her journey. Again, that's the kind of person she is. Of course, this meant she had to have another necklace.

I gave Stephanie a new one to wear while she and Tyler were awaiting their next beautiful adventure. One of the many reasons I am so passionate about this book is because so many I care about have been impacted by infertility or second infertility. It feels like an epidemic sweeping the land, not only with those whom I love but throughout the entire world. I have seen and experienced firsthand the pain that comes with infertility and loss, over and over.

I have helped wipe away many tears, prayed many prayers, given many shots, cried alongside my Sisterhood friends, shared in several awful phone calls, made numerous hospital visits, and unfortunately, have attended many memorial services for sweet angel babies. Through each experience, my heart hurt in a way I can't describe, and I yearned to do something, to help in some tangible way. Obviously, the necklace is just a piece of the puzzle. As more of those I love continue to be affected by infertility and bereavement, the more necklaces must be shared, which means this powerful Sisterhood of faith grows continually.

It became evident we could not keep these beautiful journeys to ourselves. We had to share with the world that there is this Sisterhood, a family here, standing in faith, ready and willing to encourage and welcome others to a community of hope.

I felt God call me to be the vessel to share the story of the necklace, so I reached out to more of my closest friends and family whom I had given necklaces to, those willing to impart their experiences with the world. Each story as incredible as the next.

With that being said, it is my great pleasure and honor to introduce you to Alicia, or as my kids call her, "Auntie Alicia!" We have been close friends for over fifteen years— growing up together through the different seasons of life. We have been through the best of times and the worst of times but always remaining "sisters!" It would appear God blessed us with each other for a lifetime of friendship and support, and I am incredibly thankful for that. Alicia and her sweet husband, Jason, are the kind of people you can call at 3:00 a.m., and they would be there for you in a flash! They are kind and generous, always willing to help others—and they do! They truly love children, a fact that's apparent if you were to ask all their nieces and nephews!

Therefore, when she told me they were moving forward with in-vitro fertilization, I was ecstatic. I know without a shadow of doubt, they are going to be amazing, loving parents!

This is their journey with IVF.

4

Meet Alicia

Trust in the Lord

Davis IVF Journey

I had resigned from a fifteen-year career in the auto industry. I had worked for an amazing company and had the career I always dreamed of. Jason and I were ready to grow our family and, somehow, knew now was the time. Jason had been ready for babies the second we were engaged. I was thirty-four years old and decided it was now or never. I resigned in 2016, which was one of the hardest decisions in my life to make. During 2016, we focused on getting myself back to me. I had been working thirteen-hour days with hardly any time for anything else.

We tried to conceive for fifteen months. With each monthly period also came a bit of disappointment. We prayed nonstop over my belly, day and night, asking God to guide our footsteps in the baby-making journey. I used ovulation predictor kits, which all worked great. I tested positive for ovulation every month. I kept thinking to myself, what are we missing? Is there more to this than a simple knowing when ovulation occurs? We ended up buying an ovulation bracelet, which was supposed to pinpoint ovulation even more accurately. (By no means did it do anything different than the over-the-counter ovulation kits.) We knew God was always working behind the scenes in our daily life. We trust in Him always and trusted there was a reason for all this.

We decided to contact the OB (obstetrician-gynecologist) to determine if there was something they could do to help us. We went in for a series of tests. They tested Jason's sperm, (we won't discuss how Jason felt during that process), did a whole blood panel on me, and the final test was a called a hysterosalpingogram. Those who have had that procedure done, know how extremely painful it is!

All tests came back normal, so the OB said she wanted to send us to a fertility clinic for further research. She stated that the fertility companies have more tools in their toolboxes to help narrow down fertility issues. She gave us two options to choose from and told us to take some time to find out which one would be the best match.

After much research and prayer, we decided on the fertility company we were going to go with. Let's call it, "The Center." We had read tremendous reviews, specifically about one particular doctor and felt God had led us there, exactly where he wanted us.

We had to do most blood tests all over again. The final blood test was an egg health test. Who knew an egg health test was done by blood? Pretty fascinating.

On February 22, 2018 at 2:41 p.m., our life was forever changed. We heard the news that my egg health was a .3.

For a thirty-four-year-old woman, egg health should be a 2.3.

My resting follicle count was an "8," and it should be "15–20" for my age. I dropped to the floor and cried out to God. The tears wouldn't stop for hours. I didn't know how to look Jason in the eyes and tell him that I couldn't give him babies. I couldn't give him his heart's desire. He wanted to be a daddy more than anything.

I didn't call Jason that moment to give him the news. I couldn't pull myself together enough to tell him. Jason came home from work to find me on my knees in our bedroom. He asked what happened. I explained the results to him. He grabbed me and hugged me tightly. He kept saying, "We're going to get through this. Everything will turn out exactly how God intends."

For the first time in our four years of marriage, I didn't trust what he was telling me. Had the results been reversed, Jason would have felt the same way, as if he was hurting me.

What was next?

Where do we go from here?

How do I come to terms with the fact that I can't have babies?

My heart was broken. Too broken to see the devastation on Jason's face.

Does God want me to just be the world's best auntie and Jason the world's best uncle? My sister has two beautiful babies—our nephew who is now eight and our niece who is nearly four. We have the most amazing time with them. Is this everything we get to experience? My mom had my sister and me, and my sister has two babies . . . and I can't have any?

How did this happen?

Did I do something wrong?

Was it all the bad decisions I made in my twenties?

Why, why, why?

I believe God grew tired of hearing me say "why" so many times.

Philippians 4:13 tells me, "I can do all things through Christ who gives me strength." I ask for strength every day and for God to help me keep my eyes focused on Him. Surely, I can find the strength to figure out our next steps.

If God can give up His one and only Son to die for my sins, I can surely pull it together and be open to where God is taking us.

One thing was for sure: our amazing support system and our faith are what kept us going. Jason had been my rock through this, and I couldn't push through without him. My family and friends showed us an outpouring of love during this time. They kept me spiritually alive, knowing we were right where God wanted us. I am so thankful for all my friendships. I have God to thank for those in my life.

We met with our nurse who laid out our options. She told us, excitedly, the doctor had a plan! *Praise, Jesus!*

The doctor recommended one cycle of IUI, and if that didn't take, go straight to IVF. Due to my ovarian reserve, we didn't have time to try more than one IUI. Tears of joy came over me as we sat there listening to our game plan. Thank you, Jesus, for always working behind the scenes.

My BFF, Nicole Wood, gave me my mustard seed necklace. She had given one to another friend who had gone through her own fertility journey a couple years before, and she gave that necklace to another friend going through her journey. This necklace had been passed to so many incredible godly women, all going through the same thing Jason and I were faced with. We prayed over my necklace before putting it around my neck, and I prayed over my necklace every morning after that when I put it on.

March 6, 2018 started our crazy exciting journey. I had two follicles: one measuring twenty-three millimeters and the other measuring twenty-four. They only needed to be eighteen millimeters in size, so we were thrilled knowing I had viable follicles.

As I lay in the procedure room, feet resting in stirrups, I grabbed for my necklace around my neck and prayed for our miracle. As the nurse inserted Jason's sperm, I couldn't help but become emotional. As tears rolled down my face, I noticed Jason's eyes filling with tears, and we prayed.

Then, we waited! The sperm had been implanted.

On March 14th, I had a sharp pain in my lower abdomen while I was out walking our first "daughter," Dakota. She's our precious German short hair pointer, whom we love more than words can say. By the time we had gotten warmed up, I was hunched over, not knowing if I would be able to make it back. The pain was excruciating. We were three miles away from home.

I pushed through and made it home after over an hour and called my nurse to let her know what was happening. She told me it would be too early to find out if we had suffered from an ectopic pregnancy or not. It was too early to find out anything, but the only thing to do was go in for an ultrasound to see if any cysts had popped up or not.

I chose to go in for the ultrasound just to be sure. The ultrasound was normal, no cysts.

March 20, 2018 marked fourteen days since the IUI. I took an at-home pregnancy test, which came back negative. I went in for the blood test, to confirm the negative result and sure enough, that was negative, as well.

I cried for hours, wondering why God seemed to be closing these doors. Where is He pushing us?

We met with our nurse immediately after the negative blood test to begin the IVF journey.

As we sat in those office chairs, unscrambling the numbers, the fees for our upcoming Plan *B*, we looked at each other but had no words. Costs ranged from $6,000–8,000 for the medications and $19,500 for the IVF procedure.

This did not include the hundreds of dollars we'd already spent on all the blood work, egg health medication, and the cost of the IUI.

Our health insurance did not cover any fertility treatments (as many don't), so we were left to pay out-of-pocket. There were financing options available, which the nurse went over as we secretly wondered if this was the right option for us.

We left with our packet and prayed nonstop. Jason and I decided that if we couldn't pay for it out-of-pocket, then we wouldn't go down this path. We didn't want to finance a baby, and we didn't want to go into debt to conceive. We knew all our trust had to be in God and Him alone. If we were going to do this, then Jason said he'd have to work extra hard and run leads to pay for this baby. Jason had worked hard his whole life. He owns a construction company, which God has blessed us tremendously with through the years.

We decided to go all in. This was our dream, our hearts' desire—to have babies and grow our family. It was then God unveiled some of His purpose for me—why God had led us to this point. I needed to educate women about egg health.

It's a simple blood test that identifies your egg quality and the ultrasound identifies your resting follicle count. Doctors don't know what causes your eggs' health to diminish or at what age they start their decline. A few forty-year-old women have the eggs of a twenty-year-old and some twenty-year-olds have the egg health of a fifty-year-old woman.

I believed I was being led to start a foundation to help others financially afford these hefty fertility bills. God had blessed us financially, making a way for us to pay our IVF journey. I wanted to do the same for others.

Jason and I had to do so much blood work to just start the IVF journey. We both took the Karyotyping test, which cost $213 each, and a chromosome test, which was another $200. We both had to do the infectious disease test, as well. We chose to take the genetic testing to ensure my eggs and his sperm would take.

Praise Jesus, all screening tests came back normal!

My protocol was to spend two and a half months getting my egg health up. We started the egg health protocol at the end of March.

I had to drink an ovarian reserve drink twice daily and take 75 mg of DHEA twice daily and 300 mg of CoQ10, two pills once daily. My Vitamin D levels were extremely low, so I was on a 50,000 IU of Vitamin D for eight weeks. Then, the dosage went down to 5,000 IU daily. My blood was drawn every two weeks to check all my levels to be sure they were where the doctor wanted them to be.

Weight gain from the supplements was hard on me, emotionally. I felt so bloated; my pants wouldn't button. I wanted to wear workout clothes every day and be in an oversized shirt. I told myself it would all be worth it for our end result, which hopefully would be a beautiful, healthy baby.

As we approached the end of the egg health protocol, I was placed with my amazing IVF nurse—an angel. God knew we needed her.

She set up our three-hour IVF class for June 13, 2018. This would be the class where we went over IVF in detail, learned about the embryo, and learned how to administer the injections.

On May 14, our IVF nurse mentioned a pill called Metformin and how it had changed the fertility world. It's what people with diabetes use to help metabolize sugars. Well, the other benefit of Metformin is egg health. This wasn't a make or break line item in my IVF protocol, but if it could help my chances of conceiving, then we thought, "Why not?" I wanted to do everything I could to increase our chances of having a healthy baby.

The biggest side effects of taking Metformin is stomach cramping, nausea, and diarrhea, unless you follow a very low carb diet. Everyone who knows me knows I love carbs and sweets. Mexican food, pizza, bread, crackers, desserts, chocolate . . . the list goes on. I would have to be on Metformin up until the egg retrieval date and possibly until the egg transfer. So I sacrificed.

I started Metformin May 24th. Oh, my goodness—it was a struggle to eat a low-carb diet. But I knew it'd all be worth it for the result.

June 13th was the date of our IVF class. I felt so overwhelmed. There were several other couples, all with their own fertility obstacle. I wondered, "Can I do this mentally and physically?" Shots twice daily, continued CoQ10 and Metformin, plus all other supplements that are required once injections start. Jason and I quickly became IVF experts.

The injections started June 27th, and go up until my egg retrieval, which was scheduled for July 11th or 12th. The injections help produce as many follicles as possible in the hope of promoting the viability of healthy, mature eggs inside them. Since I only had eight resting follicles, I wouldn't be at risk of having fifteen to twenty-five follicles come egg retrieval.

As way of explaining the rest of the process, once the egg retrieval happens, the team washes the sperm and looks at them to separate the abnormal and normal ones. Then they fertilize the eggs from the retrieval. Twenty-four hours later, couples know how many eggs are actually fertilized. They then go through a series of tests. They need to make it to the sixth day of testing. Once they reach day six, they are sent for biopsy. When the results come back from biopsy, they freeze the viable, normal ones and ready them for transfer.

After the egg retrieval, women spend the next month doing what's called a washout month. I cleansed my body of all supplements and meds. The second month is reserved for prepping the uterus. When all goes according to plan, the egg transfer happens; for us, that was October 2018.

What if when the egg retrieval comes, and I don't have enough eggs.

What if out of the eggs that do come out, only one makes it?

What if that one that does make it doesn't take during the transfer?

Then I'll have to do the whole egg retrieval process all over again to try and get more eggs!

I allow the spirit of fear to consume my mind. But then I feel the mustard seed necklace hanging from my throat.

My God is bigger than statistics and bigger than the Enemy. God had already won this battle. I knew He was already at the egg retrieval appointment and all nurses and embryologists would be amazed at how many healthy eggs they retrieved, even when my stats predict otherwise. My God is One of earthly statistics.

We prayed for a miracle baby, and I knew God would never leave us nor forsake us. The devil wanted me to believe his lies. Just like Mamma Marcia said: "False evidence appearing real." The devil has no place in this family!

Life and death are in the power of the tongue. I knew I had to confess our miracle daily and speak it into existence. This victory was ours!

The pharmacy called. They would be mailing me all the meds. They informed me of my total cost—$9,875. My heart stopped! *What?*

"$9,875.00?"

"Um, are you sure?" I asked. The woman confirmed it. I told her to hold on for a minute while I looked to see if I could find any coupons. I called my nurse and asked her why (in the world!) our medication bill was so high. She said it was all due to the amount of meds needed for the best possible outcome. So I shopped around. I found another fertility medication company, which listed one of the prescriptions for a bit less money. I called and ordered one medication with the other company and waited to see what else I could do.

I received a call a couple of days later from the account manager at the pharmacy that oversees patients at The

Center. She told me the previous woman had misquoted the cost because she didn't know I was a part of The Center. The accurate total was $6,795.00.

Praise Jesus! That was more like it. I bought all the meds, ordered right in time to be delivered the same day I was to start all the injections.

The day before I started my first injections, I looked at the woman I had become in the mirror, a woman who had discovered she had poor egg quality and an extremely low ovarian reserve. I've grown so much in this journey already. I'm stronger and wiser about my fertility and reproductive health. Every storm becomes beautiful and my faith became stronger.

I started the Estrace, which I must take up until my next period. I feel so nervous—scared, really—about the injections. I wondered if I'd be able to administer them by myself or if Jason would have to do it? He's the calm one. Of course, he is. He's my perfect!

I had to take four shots every day. My sister had to give me my first injection since my medication package was delivered late. She almost passed out! It took us forty-five minutes to administer the first shot. Good grief!

Jason administered all shots going forward. I had to give myself just a few for a couple of days, so that wasn't too bad. They stung but that's was it. I endured shots for twelve days.

I had to go for blood work and ultrasounds every day. They monitored each follicle. Each day, they grew. On Tuesday July 10th, my left side had five follicles. Their measurements in millimeters were: 19,16,14,13, and another 13. My right side had five follicles as well: an 18, 16, 15, 13 and a 12 mm. We had ten full-sized follicles, ready for retrieval.

We were notified on Wednesday, July 11th that we would "pull the trigger" that tonight! Woo Hoo! Both nervous and excited, I paced our house. I was ready for all the shots to end and all the daily blood work and ultrasounds to be finished.

My IVF Trigger and Pre-Op Instructions were intense. My retrieval physician was Dr. O'Shaughnessy. When we learned this at the clinic, I couldn't stop crying. My stepdad, Brian, who had passed away five years before this . . . his last name was O'Shaughnessy. I cried out to God, thanking him for being with me every step of the way. I knew my dad was right there with me, too. There couldn't have been more of a confirmation that we were where God wanted us to be.

Wednesday night was the big trigger shot in the upper, outer side of my butt muscle, along with another four shots.

Thursday morning, I endure just one shot. *Praise, Jesus!*

Every hour that passed, my anxiety about the retrieval grew. The only other time I had ever been put under anesthesia was when I had my tonsils removed at nineteen years old, and Brian had been there with me.

Retrieval Day arrived

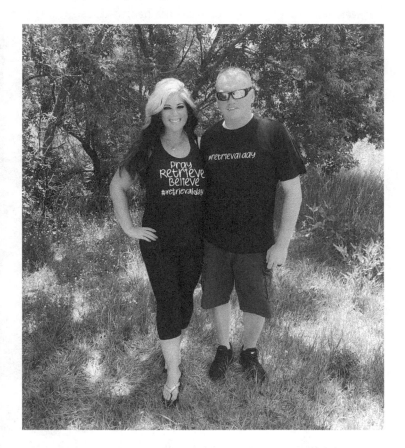

My heart beat out of my chest the whole way to The Center. I have no idea what to expect. We sat, waiting to be called for thirty minutes. The anxiety and the worry of the waiting was awful. I finally got called back to meet with the anesthesiologist. My bottom lip quivered as my eyes filled with tears. I confessed to the anesthesiologist that I was scared. He told me to relax, that I was in great hands. He was wonderful. I answered all his health questions and was deemed ready. He put heart monitors on my chest and the IV into my hand, even as the tears rolled down my face. Dr. O'Shaughnessy walked in the room, and I burst into a loud, ugly cry as I tried to explain to Dr. O'Shaughnessy about Brian and how I knew God was there in the room. Then, I don't remember anything! I was out!

I woke up and first asked for Jason. I overheard the nurse and the anesthesiologist telling him my blood pressure was 181/111. Jason's eyes widened.

"I told you *all* that I was scared," I say meekly.

Jason turned and hugged and kissed me. We were told eight follicles were retrieved and only five of them were mature eggs. A huge part of me felt devastated, knowing we only had five eggs going into this process. Statistically, I knew only half make it to the third day; then another half usually make it to the blastocyst stage.

I harbored so much worry, causing many questions. I knew God was in control, and I knew He was with me every step of the way. I should have felt thankful that we had those five mature eggs; we could have had none. I tried to focus on that, on the fact that we had five and not zero. Then, we prayed heavily over all those eggs, prayed they'd be fertilized.

Saturday came along with my update from the embryologist. Only four fertilized out of the five. *There I go, using
"only" again.* They were put in the place where they grow
to reach the blastocyst phase. All my family and closest
friends engaged in nonstop prayer. The power of prayer is
incredible and miracles do happen!

My next update doesn't come until Monday. All I
could do from Saturday to Monday was pray. I prayed
nonstop. As I looked up from praying, I saw this:

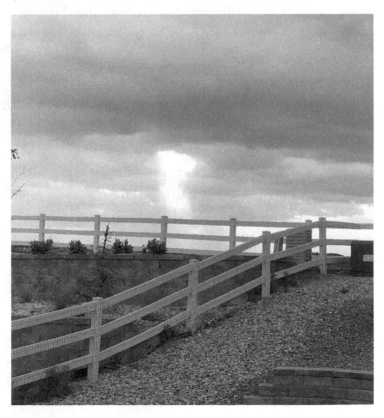

Thank you, Jesus, for never leaving me!

Monday came, and we spoke with the embryologist, three of our four embryos were at an eight-cell stage, which was right where they needed to be. *Thank you, Jesus!* Two of those were graded a "1," meaning they were the *best* they could be. The third was graded a "2," which was fair. The fourth was only at a four-cell stage and graded a "4," which is poor. They decided to wait to see if the fourth embryo would grow in the next two days. If it didn't, it would be discarded. The embryologist said the three that were at the eight-cell stage needed to keep doing what they were doing and keep growing.

We wouldn't receive another update until Wednesday. They didn't want to bother the embryos, so they were left alone until the Wednesday check.

I worried myself sick. There is power in prayer. All I could do was pray, wait, and trust. I must trust in the Lord with all my heart and know in His Will is the only place I want to be. I found myself praying with nearly every breath I took. All I could do was talk to God and try to have some sort of peace within the waiting. I reminded myself to be grateful that we had three great embryos growing, when we could have had zero reach the eight-cell stage. There were so many reasons for me to be thankful: that God has blessed Jason and me with the ability to afford this journey. I was thankful for Jason and his strength. I was thankful for the fact that we were able to play the waiting game because that meant we had embryos to wait on. I'm thankful for God's grace and mercy. His will, will be done, and I had to rest in His peace, knowing He had it all in His cupped hands.

Wednesday arrived! Sick to my stomach with the waiting, I finally get the call at the end of the day, one that told us we were going to embryo testing with two. The third embryo didn't make it. I can't control my emotions at this point. I'm so thankful that we have two going for the biopsy testing, but I had prayed and wished for that third one to have gone with the other two, so I couldn't help but feel a wee bit disappointed. "It's OK. This is God's plan."

More waiting. We're told it would take ten days to two weeks get the results back on the two sent for testing. The embryologist said that since I was thirty-four, it was in our favor. Praying now that those two both come back normal.

These next two weeks are brutal. Everything is out of my hands, and what would be, would be. I knew it was all made possible only because of God. We had trekked past all the odds. Only twenty-five to thirty percent of embryos make it to biopsy stage, and we had reached it with fifty percent of our embryos. Our God was big, and I had no words. God had laid His Hands on this journey from the very beginning. He had led us here for His reason. All we had to do was stand in agreement with Him and know we couldn't do anything else but pray, wait, and trust!

When I finally got the call from the embryologist, my heart was pounding, and I felt nauseous. I told the embryologist to hold for a second while I sat down. I asked her if it was good news or bad news. She said it was good news. I took a deep breath and started crying. She proceeded to tell me that one embryo came back normal, and the second one did not. So we have one embryo that is now frozen and ready for transfer. I asked her to not tell me the gender because I needed to hear that from Jason.

Yes, I was excited that we had the opportunity to be parents. But I couldn't help but feel robbed, causing swirling and conflicting emotions. Of course, in a perfect world, we would have two babies. Instead, we only get the possibility to be parents to one baby.

Why am I feeling so down? I feel as if my heart was ripped out once again. In the moment, I know I sounded ungrateful (even now, I feel the shame of ingratitude), but why were we robbed of having our hearts' desire? Why wouldn't God want us to have more than one baby? Thousands of questions took over my mind, and I had to shut them out.

I called Jason as soon as I hung up with the embryologist. I told him that one came back normal and the other did not. He was over the moon excited, and his voice started shaking as I heard him cry. I told him I wanted to know the gender, but I needed to hear it from him. Since we only had one, I couldn't wait any longer to find out.

So Jason called the embryologist and called me back about thirty seconds later.

"I can't be more excited to tell you . . . it's a girl!" Jason couldn't stop talking about how thrilled he was, thanking God for giving him the chance to be a daddy. All he wanted was to be a daddy. As I listen to the joy in his voice, all I can think of is that we only have one.

Jason told me to pull it together and be thankful that we had been given this one chance and to thank God for all He had done. I knew my attitude was horrible, and I did need to get it together; I just needed a moment to gather my emotions and talk to God and try to come to terms with all of it.

It took me the entire weekend to put myself back together and apologize to God for having such a bad attitude. I felt horrible that I had even felt that way. I prayed nonstop, asking God to forgive me and that I was sorry for feeling that way. I knew God had bigger plans, and I needed to once again just wait and trust in Him.

Wow, what a fighter she was to have made it through all that testing and growing. I can't begin to imagine what God has in store for our baby girl, a.k.a., Baby Grace.

A week went by and I continued to ask God for His forgiveness regarding my poor attitude and continued to thank Him in advance for a perfect transfer and for us to become pregnant.

I walked Dakota every morning. One morning, as I pulled up my iTunes for my morning walk, the song that came on was "Grace wins." *Wow!* Is God present or what? Yes, Baby Grace wins! She will make it through the transfer! I knew I had to confess it and believe it would happen!

A few days later, I received a call from my IVF nurse. She wanted to check in on me and see how everything was going. I told her that Jason and I were extremely grateful that we had one embryo, and we had a chance at becoming parents. I confessed to her we were also bummed that we only had one chance at this.

The nurse mentioned something called "embryo banking," which means we go through another month of egg health supplements, go through all the injections again, and relent to another egg retrieval to see if we can get any more. I asked her what the cost was and she stated it would be just the cost of meds plus the egg retrieval. I had a sense of hope again for the first time since we had started the journey. I told her I needed to go over it with Jason, and we would get back to her the next day. She said OK and that she would have the financial team email me the price sheet to get started. I called Jason and let him know the good news. He was on board!

"My number one concern is you. Are you up for it?" he said.

"Yes!"

Round 2! Praise Jesus, I was with Nicole and Mama Marcia that day, so they became my sounding boards. Would this be our second chance at having more than one baby? Could I physically and mentally do this all over again? Was this God's way of showing us that our dream of having two beautiful babies was here?

We could totally do this! We had the funds to make it happen with the cost of meds and the retrieval. This would mean that our transfer date would be pushed back another two months. Part of me was ready for the transfer immediately because I was so excited. But the other part of me, wanted more than one baby, so I thought we should bank now. We had just finished the injections, and going right back into it would be fine.

A few hours later, I read an email from the financial team at The Center. The email stated the IVF cost was $9,875.00, plus the cost of meds, plus the cost of the retrieval. I must have stared at the $9,875.00 for at least five minutes with no words. $9,875.00 was not what my nurse had quoted. She didn't mention anything about additional costs. I called the financial team and asked what the $9,875.00 was for and that my nurse told me it was just the cost of meds, plus the retrieval. The financial team stated my nurse had no authority to tell me that because she did not work in billing—she was wrong. The $9,875.00 was the cost of the embryo-making process, along with the IVF portion for round two. Jason and I would be responsible for the $9,875.00, plus the cost of meds, plus the retrieval. Within two seconds, I told her no. We would pass.

Once again, I felt robbed. Why were all these choices being ripped from me? Was God protecting us from something? I knew all things were possible with Him, and I knew His Will was the only good and safe place to be. So I believed He was protecting us from something. Maybe nothing would have come back this time from biopsy, and we'd still only have one.

I wait for Jason to come home before I tell him this news. As I tell him, disappointment etches across his face. "Even if we had the additional $9,875.00 right now, I still wouldn't do it. That's just ridiculous. If we only had to pay for the meds and the retrieval, then yes, I would be totally on board. But that additional cost is just too much. We just finished paying $35,000."

God answered our prayers by closing that door for us. Jason was in agreement: paying that additional cost was just not what we were going to choose. At what point, as a couple with one embryo in one basket, we surrendered gave it to God. God was ultimately in control, not us. We didn't want to try to be in control. God had a bigger plan.

I will never understand our journey, but I do know I could never have gone through this with anyone else but God and Jason.

But the support from our family and friends was more than we could have ever prayed for. I never thought I'd be the only one out of all my friends and family with fertility issues. It's a tough pill to swallow. I've come to terms with the fact that this story is what we've been given, and its up to us to make the best of it. It's how I deal with the trials and how my attitude remains stable and upbeat. Jason is the most amazing husband and godly man I know, and I'm so thankful for him. Just when I thought I couldn't possibly fall more in love with him, I did. This whole journey bonded us and lifted us to a whole new level in our marriage. I prayed fervently that I would give him his heart's desire—to be called Daddy.

The emotional roller coaster of emotions, the hours spent crying, all the devastation, and heartbreak brought me closer to God. My relationship with God grew immensely through each trial. Through Him, I found new strength and a new purpose. I'd always known my relationship with God was strong, and we had a good way of communicating with one another, but this journey brought us even closer. I'm always amazed at how God works, but He's done something different during this trial. I was pushed to places I'd never been before. I leaned on Him in more ways than I did when Brian died and when I was faced with other heartbreaking trials I'd been through. This one was different. I can't explain it right now; maybe after the transfer happens, and we have the positive pregnancy test, I'll be able to explain this feeling. To explain how God lives and flows through my blood, how I can feel His presence now, more than ever before.

****

Every time I read Alicia's story, Proverbs 3:5–6 comes to mind. "Trust in the Lord with all your heart, do not depend on your own understanding. Seek His will in all you do and He will show you which path to take."

Alicia lives her life this way. No matter what she faces, she always trusts the Lord and His will for her life. I have seen her confronted with some incredibly difficult things, and each time, she stands stronger than before as she relies on her faith. A true example of a Proverbs 31 woman!

She is an inspiration to many because she is authentic and vulnerable; she will tell you and God exactly how she feels. She may be frustrated, hurting, and questioning what's happening around her, but with each new struggle, she manages to grow closer to God and those around her. I remember talking about how this whole process could draw her and Jason closer to each other, and that's exactly what has happened. They have chosen to rely on each other and stand strong in their faith. It is incredible to see the tranquility that comes from truly seeking and trusting God. It brings calm in the midst of the storm.

Sisters, Transfer Day was a pure success! Everything went perfectly, just as the doctors—and God—had planned! Just as we had hoped and prayed for! I remember the day my sister Alicia called and told me she was, indeed, pregnant!

We cried and celebrated and thanked God for the beautiful miracle growing in her tummy! Every month that passed, we fell more and more in love with Chloe Grace!

We could not wait for her arrival, so when Alicia asked my mom and me to be in the room when she delivered her, we were honored and, of course, cried some more!

We could not imagine being anywhere else. We knew what a treasure it would be to share in this precious time with her and her family.

That day, Alicia's strength and faith were indeed tested. She had complications with her epidural, and it ended up not working. She was in a tremendous amount of pain, and something did not seem quite right. No one could figure it out, but God did. He was there in the chaos, working behind the scenes.

The time on the clock was progressing but not Alicia's delivery. After many nurses and doctors flew in and out of the room, chatting, we kept our eyes on Chloe's monitor, watching her heartbeat jump around. At one point, I scared poor Jason because I yelled something when I saw her heartbeat soar!

We all looked at each other and knew we needed God's wisdom and divine intervention. We laid hands on Alicia and prayed over her and Chloe and asked God for His direction and protection.

After another contraction and more time passing by, Alicia looked right at me. "What do you think I should do?"

In that moment, God spoke to me clearly and said these very words: "Tell Alicia not to push; she needs a C-section."

Talk about goosebumps all over your body. In those moments, repeating His words, we cried together and knew we had to listen. Alicia's beautiful mom, Kathy, informed the doctors with urgency that Alicia was ready for her C-section.

Thank God she did because when the doors finally flew open, and Jason came out to tell us Chloe was here, the whole waiting room cheered and thanked God! Another miracle! *Thank you, Jesus!*

The doctors said that if Alicia had not had a C-section, the outcome would have been very different!

In times of testing and crucial moments like these, what should we do? What do we do?

We put our faith and trust in the Lord and listen to the small still voice that speaks in our Spirit.

2 Corinthians 3:17 (NIV) says, "Now the Lord is the spirit, and where the Spirit of the Lord is, there is freedom."

John 14:16 (NIV) says, "And I will ask the Father, and he will give you another advocate to help you and be with you forever."

Every time we look at Chloe, we are reminded of God's favor and love. In fact, her middle name, Grace, means, "favor" in Hebrew. Chloe will grow up to be a world changer full of love, grace, and strength, just like her precious mommy!

Sisterhood, no matter what journey you are on, stand strong, and do not give up hope! Your miracle is just around the corner!

As I mentioned previously, my faith defines the way I live my life. Over time, it has allowed me to see life through a positive filter and given me a resilience that I might not otherwise have. My husband and I talk about people who have "happy eyes," you know the kind of people that walk around with a twinkle. You look at them and instantly feel connected; you can sense their joy and ultimately, know there is something uniquely different about them.

This connection is one I believe comes from deep within our souls. The place where we seek and receive Jesus. I bring this up because oftentimes, as a Christian counselor, I am asked questions such as, "Where does faith come from? How can I trust so blindly? Is it possible to have peace again? Can I ever be made whole? How can I be forgiven? How can I ever forgive him or her? How can I have eternal life? How do you know God is real?"

My answer always goes back to one name. The one name that changed everything—forever!

Jesus Christ.

You see, faith does not have to be complicated; it is simple.

John 3:16 (NLT) says, "For this is how God loved the world, He gave his one and only Son so that everyone who believes in him will not perish but have eternal life. God sent his son into world not to judge the world, but to save the world through Him."

And Romans 10:13 says, "For everyone who calls on the name of the Lord will be saved."

In other words, if you would like to begin a relationship with Jesus and develop a faith that can move mountains, it starts with believing that God loves you so much that He sent His son to save you from your sins. This small step of faith begins the journey. This is the same step of faith that each of these beautiful woman took to begin their hope-filled journeys.

It can be a humbling experience to admit you cannot make it on your own, that you are in need of a Savior. For me, part of wearing my mustard seed necklace was about surrender. Surrendering my fears and my unknown future to Him while standing in faith that nothing was impossible for Him. If you have faith the size of a mustard seed, it is not about you and what you can do; it becomes about Him and what He can do.

Psalm 37:5 (NIV): "Commit everything you do to the Lord. Trust Him, and he will help you."

Sisters, when we trust in Jesus and accept Him as our savior, it makes Heaven our home and all of His promises ours.

With that being said, I would like to introduce to you to my cousin, Leanne, who embodies faith, strength, courage, and hope in spite of enduring a tragedy that would cause most people to doubt God's goodness and give up the dream of parenting a child here on Earth.

5

Meet Leanne

Courage on Fire

Our story began in June 2012. My husband, Chris, and I had been together since 2004 and married for a year. We were both on the same page—ready to start a family. In June 2012, we got pregnant the first month we tried and were thrilled that it had happened so quickly. We shared the news with our families, and our hopes and dreams for this child grew daily. I was excited when I went in for my first doctor's appointment at eight weeks.

The ultrasound tech told us, "There's no movement and no heartbeat." We were told we had a fifty, fifty chance of this baby surviving; though, we might be a little too early to detect a heartbeat. Very conflicting messages for new parents-to-be.

So we went in the following week and learned conclusively the baby hadn't survived. As a woman, I felt guilt and shame and wondered what I could have done differently. I laid in bed and cried during the weeks leading up to my D&C (dilation and curettage) in August. My procedure went well, but I felt so empty and alone leaving the hospital. I couldn't understand how or why this had happened to me.

The months that followed were filled with sadness, isolation, and aloneness. As many loss mothers feel, all I wanted was to be pregnant again.

Chris and I fell pregnant again in November 2012. We were more guarded this time and asked for extra monitoring. We held our excitement at bay and waited to tell our families until after our first appointment confirmed the heartbeat. We blew out collective breaths of relief.

Shortly after, we found out we were having a girl. Chris and I had talked years before conceiving that if we had a girl, we would name her Tenley. We bought balloons and revealed the gender and name to our family. My pregnancy was pretty uneventful until the last few weeks.

At week thirty-six, I learned I had group B strep. This is a fairly common diagnosis for pregnant women. I was told we would just treat the baby before delivery, and everything would be okay.

When August 2013 hit, I felt a little off, like I had some kind of bug but didn't think much of it. I tried to get as much rest as possible. I experienced a beautiful spiritual moment in my parents' backyard during this time. It was August 2nd. I was sitting on their back porch, in the evening, when a butterfly came and sat right next to me. I thought it was rare that a butterfly would show up in the evening, sit so close to me, and stay for so long. I felt there was a purpose, or meaning, but wasn't sure what it could be at the time.

The next morning, early in the morning, I started having back pain. I have a pretty high pain tolerance, so I knew something was wrong. Chris and I headed to the hospital. The doctors took my vitals and noticed Tenley's heart was racing. I was given an epidural and told we were headed in for an emergency C-section. The doctors broke my water and noticed blood and meconium. They believed Tenley was infected with group *B* strep. When Tenley was delivered, my first awareness was that she wasn't crying. She was placed on oxygen, and the doctors worked on her. Around noon, the medical team told us they would be airlifting Tenley to another hospital with a higher-level NICU, one with the capability of performing a procedure called Ecmo. This procedure would help Tenley breathe on her own.

Once we arrived at this new hospital, we settled in and started to pray. We were in shock—terrified that our sweet baby was in this position. Tenley underwent her first procedure but began to turn purple. The Ecmo tubes had been placed in the wrong spot, so she had to go through the procedure again. The second time, the tubes were placed better, and her color got a little bit better.

As we waited for her to improve, we had Tenley baptized by my uncle, Don. During my stay in the hospital, the thoughts of the butterfly sitting next to me wouldn't escape my mind. I started to research the meaning of butterflies. I learned they symbolize transformation and joy. In Christianity, the butterfly is a symbol of the soul and reflects the need for movement from where we are to the next phase of being.

Tenley fought for her life that whole week, and on her original due date, August 8, 2013, she experienced a brain bleed. Tenley went to be with the Lord.

We were given five beautiful days with Tenley, ones filled with hope, prayers, and family members holding her. We were approached by a wonderful foundation named Now I Lay Me Down to Sleep. This is a non-profit that provides families with a photographer, free of charge, who takes photos of parents and their children in their last moments of life. My husband and I were scared, hesitant of the emotional weight of this offer, but ultimately, we accepted. We gave her a bath and washed her hair . . . and changed her diaper. A care package arrived with a beautiful white dress for her to wear. We lay with Tenley as she took her last breath. I really don't have words to express what it feels like to have your child die in your arms; it is a profound and life changing moment, laced with the deepest sorrow anyone can possibly experience. We will forever cherish the photos of Chris and I holding Tenley.

As we left the hospital without Tenley, Chris struggled to take the car seat out of the backseat. We called our neighbor to take the bassinet out of our bedroom and to shut the nursery door before we arrived home. Tenley's body was taken to the funeral home. We had a beautiful memorial for Tenley and appreciated all of the family and friends who came to celebrate her brief life.

After losing Tenley, Chris and I attended a support group for families who had lost babies. This support group offered so much healing and hope. It was comforting to know that we were not alone, and being in the presence of others, who had experienced the same pain, made it easier to cope with the emotions we were battling. We learned about the stages of grief and how men and women grieve differently. We also learned that losing a child is the most painful thing a person can go through. There is a ninety percent divorce rate for families who experience the death of a child. Chris and I refused to be another statistic. Not only did we grow closer to each other through the death of

Tenley, but over time, we would learn how our sweet girl would change our lives in the most positive of ways.

I met a gal in my support group who also lost a little girl full-term and who was also a teacher. We had many things in common, including the desire to help others. Abby McFerron approached me with an opportunity to help her start up a support group for grieving families called Denver Share. What an amazing journey we began together that day.

We were given the opportunity to run our group free of charge in the Thrive Learning Center. This space is vastly different from the hospitals and churches where the groups commonly gather. We meet on the second Wednesday of every month and have a website, www.denvershare.org. We have recently become a non-profit organization and are able to offer mala necklace making, yoga, and other grief-healing activities to our families. Through the experience of running this support group, I have been humbled and honored to learn of others' loss stories and walk alongside them in their journeys toward healing.

During the time Abby and I started our Denver Share Chapter, Chris and I continued to try for another baby. We tried for a year without success. We started seeing fertility doctors. We underwent two IUIs, becoming pregnant both times. Unfortunately, we miscarried both babies in the first trimester.

But we refused to give up and had a third IUI. We got pregnant, and this time, we had a heartbeat! This baby was growing—on track and without any concerns—and we thought we were in the clear after our first trimester ended. Sometime within my fifteenth week of pregnancy, I began to bleed. I thought it might be due to the stress and sadness I typically feel when we flip to August on the calendar. The month holds so many difficult memories.

I went to the doctor on the anniversary of Tenley's birthday, August 3, and our fifteen-week-old baby girl did not have a heartbeat. I started contracting on my way home from work on August 4th and delivered her at home. We had testing done and were told she had an extra 13th chromosome, and ultimately, she wouldn't have been able to survive. My husband and I decided we would try IVF as our last ditch effort to give birth to a healthy child.

We started the IVF process, and there were endless tests, but we knew we'd have to be patient. Until this point, we really hadn't found any answers to our struggles. My previous doctors had been baffled by my medical history and chart, as nothing could be connected with our five losses.

We met with Dr. William Schoolcraft. In my opinion, he is one of the smartest people I have ever met. He told Chris and me that we had slightly low egg quality and that our best shot at having a living child would be with IVF—specifically with ICSI (a type of sperm injection) and chromosomal testing through a frozen cycle. We were on board and took out a line of credit on our home to cover the cost of the IVF.

We retrieved eleven eggs, nine were fertilized, and two grew to day five. Of the two embryos that grew to day five, only one of them was normal after the chromosomal testing. We knew this was our one last shot.

My IVF transfer went well and was performed on the day my grandfather, Jerome, passed. I found out the pregnancy was viable and progressing on the day of his funeral. My pregnancy with Sloane, the name we gave to our growing daughter, was filled with both fear and hope. I had a hard time connecting with her. As a loss mama, I didn't want any kind of pregnancy announcement or baby shower. Those events were, and still are, a source of pain, which I don't think will ever go away. On the morning of November 16, 2016, my grandfather appeared in my dream as a younger version of himself. He was dressed in white and was so happy, waving to me with a smile.

That next morning, I went in for what turned out to be my last doctor's appointment. I did not pass my nonstress test and was sent to the hospital. I was treated for group B strep and was about to have a C-section, eight hours after my arrival. Fear erupted in deep places.

My husband and I had connected over the last year finding pennies and dimes. They had become sweet signs of Tenley. When we left our waiting room, Chris found a dime on the floor and smiled because we knew that Tenley was there in spirit and would watch over us during the birth of Sloane. After reflecting on the dream I had that morning and the crucial dates Sloane was conceived, I couldn't help but think my grandfather had watched over my pregnancy and was watching over the birth of Sloane.

Our sixth pregnancy was the charm and our sweet rainbow baby was born—alive and well!

As soon as I stopped breastfeeding Sloane, my husband and I wanted to attempt a new cycle of IVF to see if we could have another living child. We started the testing process and discovered we were already eight weeks pregnant.

Initially, we were shocked because I hadn't been pregnant naturally since Tenley, and we were also scared we might miscarry again. We had a heartbeat and completed the genetic testing. To our surprise, everything was perfect. Our genetic results showed we were awaiting our miracle boy, to be born in August 2018.

I lose my breath a little every time August comes around. It is a month that brought us Tenley and two other sweet babies, whom we had to say good-bye to. I believed God wanted to reward us for our perseverance and also teach us that we should never lose faith.

Many loss parents report sadness and difficulty with their pregnancies and raising their rainbow babies. It is a hard thing to learn that even though you have a living child, the pain and the sadness you feel as you think of your child who passed—and the milestones they are missing—will never go away.

Strangely, loss parents do not necessarily want that sadness to go away. We know that grief is love, and we will never stop thinking about, or loving, our children in Heaven. We want to speak about our children, not for attention but for the sole purpose of honoring their existence, of acknowledging they still matter.

The biggest gift you can give a loss parent is to say their child's name. Tenley has impacted my life in a profound way. She has changed the person I am to the core. I am more empathetic and aware that everyone has their own cross to bear. My cross to bear happened to be infertility and recurrent loss. Everyone has a journey and a story. I am so blessed that Tenley and my four other losses are part of my story.

Thinking back over the years of my story, I realize how many families have been impacted by Tenley's life and death. My mother, Rhonda Bates, and I have volunteered for Now I Lay Me Down to Sleep to make hundreds of care packages for families who lose babies in local Colorado hospitals. My mother has crocheted countless blankets and hats for these care packages. Our families regularly attend the Walk to Remember put on by Now I Lay Me Down to Sleep. The proceeds from the walk go toward the creation of these care packages and the photography we were blessed to receive in the hospital.

I have co-lead Denver Share Support Group for the last three years. I will be taking a break from co-leading the group in August to, God-willing, take care of the baby we are expecting. Throughout the year, I complete random acts of kindness in memory of my babies. I hope to continue to spread awareness and offer empowerment to families impacted by loss, recurrent loss, infertility, IVF, and high-risk pregnancies.

Thank you for reading my story.

****

Sisterhood, talk about courage on fire!

Swallowing the lump in the back of my throat is nearly impossible when I read my sweet cousin's story; she and Chris are real-life superheroes, if you ask me. Their strength, desire, courage, and determination are beyond empowering. They are some of the strongest people you could ever meet. To say that I admire them and their exquisite hearts is an understatement.

If you ever have the delightful opportunity of meeting Leanne, you will see exactly why she is the perfect person to help lead a support group. Her heart and passion for life flow into a kindness that is rare and contagious. She has taken all of her painful experiences and used them to help serve others in their times of need and suffering. She and her family are continually paying it forward!

Her journey, although filled with sorrow, is also one filled with joy, faith, and miracles! From the butterflies to the most incredible update!

Megaphone and drumroll please . . .

It is with the greatest honor I announce that their precious son, Cooper, was born—picture-perfect, beautiful, and healthy in every way!

I get chills and cry each time I think of him, their going in to start the IVF process, and the discovery of their gorgeous baby boy, who was already there, already knit into his beautiful mother's womb, and then born in the month of August.

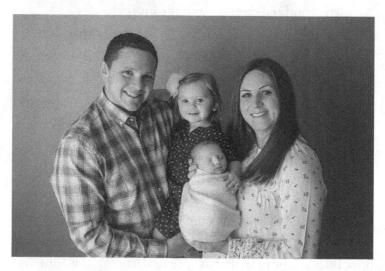

Whew—that is a powerful testimony to God's goodness! A living, breathing miracle!

The definition of a miracle is a surprising and welcome event that is not explicable by natural or scientific laws and is therefore considered to be the work of a divine agency.

We are surrounded by miracles every day and everywhere! Remember to look for them and remind yourself that with God, all things are possible!

We honor and remember precious Tenley and the impact she has made on this world.

Her legacy lives on in so many ways; through her amazing family, through every act of kindness shared, through each support group meeting, through every walk, and within each memorial event. We still experience special reminders of her life and, of course, will say her name with every butterfly we see! She is in our hearts forever, along with the rest of our beautiful angel babies.

Being surrounded by truly remarkable and kind people is a gift and one of life's greatest blessings. Oftentimes, I am overwhelmed with gratitude and can't stop thanking God for my family and friends. Some would say I am lucky, but I don't believe in luck; I call it being blessed. I know how fortunate I am to walk through life with these extraordinary people as God leads the way.

With that being said, I would like to introduce you to another sister in this Sisterhood—Katie. She is now your friend even though you may not know her. That is the kind of person she is. To know her is to love her.

I remember serving homeless people together at an event in downtown Denver. As we were passing out food and clothes, I literally saw Katie give someone the shirt off her back. In fact, I believe it was a very nice football jersey that she so freely gave away with a huge smile on her face.

Her heart is made of gold and her home is full of love. I am so thankful to call Katie and her husband, Jordan, our friends. Our husbands have been close for years, so we have truly shared life together, and it has been pure joy, through the happy times and even the dark ones because shared love and support is a genuine treasure.

When I asked Katie to share their story, I felt a tad bit selfish. No, let's be honest . . . very selfish. Because they are still in a whirlwind of busyness. However, the account of their youngest son Judah's life is one that had to be shared with the world. He is indeed a miracle and a constant reminder of God's faithfulness, like a rainbow after the storm.

This is their story.

6

Meet Katie

Judah's Journey—The Rainbow After the Storm

The eerily silent room folded in on itself. My world stopped, even as I watched everyone moving around me. I was stuck down, drowning in a nightmare that had stolen my breath from the very lungs that gave me life.

I've never had two opposing emotions happen nearly simultaneously, nor ones that stung so badly. I felt nail-biting excitement when the day finally arrived to see that precious baby again and they pulled up the monitors. Then

I experienced such heart-crushing, bone-chilling silence and horror in the next minutes.

Just two weeks before, we had seen the tiny flicker of our precious baby's heart, a joy that has no words. Then, the picture was still, the room was spinning, and I felt like I was exploding from within. All I could do was hold my husband's hand and feel the hot tears that wouldn't stop flowing. My heart would never be the same. Pieces were stolen from me, and I know I can't get them back.

The weeks that followed weren't any easier. I walked through life in slow motion, but everything around me seemed to move in fast-forward. I was constantly reminded of the emptiness I felt inside. I had lost an incredible job as a vessel, left gutted and with no purpose. I lived angry, confused, and dazed.

My body used to be an incredible tool, full of energy, health, and hope. With this event, I viewed my body as a broken failure that couldn't protect my baby. My eyes burned from reading up on all the maybes and tips and sad stories of others losses. I wouldn't wish the pain of miscarriage on my worst enemy. Life changed; I had to figure out where to go from this pit. I didn't have that safe feeling of happiness, but instead, I developed a guarded view on life. I knew God had been with me, and I knew He had forgiven me of my anger toward Him. I'm only human, and my grief brought a dark time in my life. My world had been shaken, and I needed time to heal. Even in my time of despair and anguish, I knew we were meant to have six kids this side of Heaven.

With the most recent miscarriage, I felt so selfish even thinking that. I had already been blessed with five beautiful children. I felt guilty that others struggled to even have one, and there I was, obsessing over my five losses. I will forever love all five of my babies, all five who now rest in Heaven. The only thing that kept me fighting was my knowing I served a God of miracles, and He had made it clear in my heart—I was meant to have one more on earth.

I've had times in my life where I followed the Holy Spirit's calling, unwavering even in the midst of chaos and confusion. But this most recent miscarriage took the cake. I felt partially insane, or maybe I was just making everything up in my head. How can God really want me to have one more even after five heartbreaking losses? My first son was born when I was extremely young. I had the innocence of pregnancy back then. Not worrying about every little symptom or non-symptom. I lacked the knowledge of what a true miracle pregnancy and birth is—to hold life inside myself and deliver someone. That innocence and sheer oblivion was stolen after our first loss. I had felt heart-broken for friends who had lost babies, but until I experienced the pain myself, I had no idea how incredibly difficult it is. Now, when I hear about friends—or even people I don't know—losing a baby, my heart breaks all over again for them.

In the following years, I swore every time we lost another baby that I was done. I couldn't possibly have more of my heart ripped away; I didn't think it was even possible. I didn't think I'd have any heart left. Yet each time we suffered, we persevered. It wasn't pretty, not even remotely so. It was downright ugly. It was raw. I told myself to not get excited when I saw those two lines each time.

"After all, how long will this last this time?" I was cynical. "How on earth could God let our hearts be ripped out so many times if this was truly His Will?"

I didn't know how to show my pain when I was already so blessed with my children here on earth. The emotions just about made me crazy. No that's wrong . . . they for sure made me crazy. Looking into my sweet husband's eyes during the trials was the hardest. I knew he was holding it in and trying to be strong for me. He felt led by the Holy Spirit that we were going to have one more. He said he knew it would be a boy, and even had a name. He never wavered, not once, in any of it. His heart broke right along with mine, but he always kept strong for our family and me. When we found ourselves with our last loss, I promised I would exhaust every route before I decided to let it go. But I was starting to crumble and wanted to let go of hope.

The doctor couldn't determined the reason why we were going through secondary infertility, the struggle to conceive and give birth after already having had children.

We would get incredible numbers back with the testing, see those sweet hearts beating on the screen, only to have them stop in the weeks that followed. Nothing feels as silent and lonely as looking at your perfect little baby floating lifelessly inside you with perfect little fingers, perfect little toes.

We decided to take the next step and visit a fertility specialist. We made an appointment with a doctor who could see us within a month. I wanted to know if I was going to put this dream to rest or keep pushing forward. My tank was running empty, but I knew I had to give it everything I possibly could.

Our first appointment felt like the first day of school when I was a kid, thinking of all the possible ways it could go wrong. We were anxious, excited, and scared. She was very thorough, went over all the testing we would have done, and reassured us they would exhaust every avenue. They typed up a plan, and we went over to the lab to take our first blood tests. Again, that doubt crept in: "They would think I'm selfish for seeking treatment for another baby when we were already blessed."

Satan had a hay day with me the entire journey, and some days, I let him win. It's not something I'm proud of, but it's the truth. I'm only human. That's what I love most about God; He really is like a father. Full of grace and mercy, loving us even when we don't deserve it. Forgiving us even when we are angry. I felt unworthy of another blessing, felt silly putting myself and my family through the pain. The self-doubt was nothing more than a lie. God had good plans for us, plans He made sure we felt in our hearts and souls. Plans He stood by for every heartbreaking and joyous step we took.

I was at the gym when I received the first phone call with results. I sat in the car and listened to a message telling me to call them back. I was so excited. "Yes, they found what is wrong with me!" Who would ever have thought I'd be joyous to find something wrong, yet there I was. My heart was thumping through my chest, and I begged my younger kids to please be quiet while I made a phone call. The doctor answered and told me it seemed I had a blood-clotting disorder, but that she was confident it shouldn't be causing my miscarriages. However, she was glad to find it so I could be treated during the next pregnancy.

My fifth miscarriage resulted in a D & C procedure. I had taken pills to let my body do it naturally, but after five rounds of pills, my body would not let go of the baby, and I had to schedule the surgery. Even though my baby had passed away, it was still holding on. The new doctor thought that was probably why I had the blood results come back with an abnormality. She recommended following up with a hematologist after a few weeks to see if they were still abnormal. I was disappointed; the hope slowly flew away again. I was certain they would have found concrete answers for me, but here we were once again with nothing solid to go on. I became angry again. In fact I turned up the music so my girls couldn't hear, and then I started yelling at God.

"Why would you put something so strong on my heart and then keep dragging me through the crud?"

We got home and my heart felt a tug. There He was again, the Holy Spirit, assuring me to keep going and hold on. I was in the palm of His Hand. My anger turned into sorrow, and I blasted the song "I Will Praise You in This Storm" by Casting Crowns. I was singing at the top of my lungs. I'm sure our neighbors didn't appreciate my sobbing ugly-cry singing, but I knew God loved every second of it. And He sent peace over me. So I decided to hold on a little longer. I made a phone call and set up yet another appointment—this time with the hematologist.

A few weeks later, I went for my appointment to get a HSG and an ultrasound done at the fertility clinic. Every time I walked in there, I prayed over the women I saw. I didn't know their stories, and I didn't have to. When you lose a child or have a hard time keeping a pregnancy or even getting pregnant, you're automatically a part of a club you never wanted to be a part of. I knew there were hurting hearts all over that building. Each one on their own journey, each one pushing through tests and needles and medicines with a glimmer of hope for the future.

I was praying my way through when my name was called. I had my ultrasound first. The tech was extremely nice and asked me if I had recently had surgery. I told her about my D & C, but it had been over two months ago. She seemed concerned but smiled and told me the procedure was over, and I could go next door for my next test. I walked over and immediately got called for the HSG, so I went back and jumped on the table, and they started to inject the ink. The lady's face was puzzled. I thought it must just be my nerves or the fact that I have a really long cervix. I've had all C-sections because of this, and it was nothing new to me. She showed me the pictures and asked if I wanted to take a picture with my phone. I declined, thinking it was weird she asked me. I got dressed and was relieved it was over with and went on my way.

It wasn't ten minutes later that I got a call from the doctor. She sounded panicked and asked me if I could come back in and take an HCG test to make sure I wasn't pregnant. I laughed, thinking, "Lady, I hope I am, but I know I'm not!" She said if I was, it was life threatening. Again, there I sat dumbfounded at the news. So I made a U-turn, illegally, and raced off.

I pulled into the clinic and forced myself to get out of the car. I was sweating profusely from the anger that had been unleashed inside me. An innocent test had turned into a living nightmare.

"God, where the heck are you?"

Was I just making it up in my head that we've felt led to another child? I was so certain that God was the only

One who could have put this in my heart. And yet here I was doubting, lost, and feeling forgotten. Something inside made me open up that car door and place both feet on the ground. It was as if I was walking in a dream. I had felt this way several times in my journey, like I wasn't the one in the driver's seat, and yet my body kept moving forward. Looking back at those feelings, I know for certain God was carrying me through. At the time, I didn't want to give any credit to Him because of my breaking, stubborn heart. He still held me, though, and kept me moving.

I had been through five heart-breaking losses: hemorrhaged on my son's field trip, labored with each baby, lost sleep, experienced loss of faith, and felt sheer sorrow. Surely if He got me through those days, He would get me through this setback.

They took my blood, and I was on my way back home. The sun shown through the driver-side window, and for a second, I closed my eyes and felt the goodness of its rays. Better days are ahead; I am not forgotten.

The doctor called back within an hour to let me know I was indeed "not pregnant" and to make sure to keep it that way. They scheduled me an appointment and halted our testing for the time being.

When the day of the appointment came, my rock of a husband was right there with me. It never mattered what he had going on or what he felt through this journey, he was always there by my side. It was a miracle I was blind to when the pain took over. God had blessed me with such an incredible life partner. We walked hand-in-hand into the clinic, prepared for whatever was to come. Or so we thought.

The doctor sat us down and pulled up my test images on the computer screen. We had no idea what we were looking at, nor did it matter. We knew for certain God was ordering our footsteps, and that's what we had to keep doing, taking steps. She broke the news to us that our journey to get pregnant was over. Something we didn't expect or accept. I sat in silence. She said we could do surrogacy as an option, but that if we got pregnant, I would die, as may our baby.

She diagnosed me with a C-section scar dehiscence. My scar was opening up from the inside out. The images on the tests showed the ink leaking out of my uterus, something they had never seen before. She had a meeting with the other doctors in the practice, and they all agreed. We asked if I could have surgery to fix it. We were given another answer we didn't want to hear. This condition was rare and usually only happened when people were pregnant and their uterus had grown, causing the tear. We left pretty shaken and baffled. Yet there was my husband, again reminding me that we serve a God who does the impossible every day. Reminding me that though the doctor's report said one thing, God says something else.

After spending some time processing and peeling back the many layers of emotions I was going through, I dug in. I exhausted every avenue to get to our miracle baby. We would one day be telling our story to encourage others to keep fighting when the world says no but they know God says yes. I got on my computer and spent hours researching my condition and ways to fix it. There wasn't a lot I could find, and even though it was discouraging, I wasn't going to let that discouragement beat me. Like the saying goes, "You can knock me down, but I'm going to keep getting up." I felt a peace that if God wanted this to happen, it would and if not, at least I knew I did everything I could. I emailed and called dozens of doctors who had done surgeries like the one I thought I needed. Essentially, it would be like having another C-section to fix it, and after already having five of those, it wasn't ideal.

Ideal was never a part of this equation though. After a few weeks and countless hours trying to get answers, I found myself emailing my ob-gyn. I figured I would just keep him in the loop of all the things we had been up to and the test results I had been given. That same day, he sent an email back with some of the best news we had ever received. One of the doctors in their practice specialized in robotic surgery. He was willing to do the surgery for us! I made an appointment with him, feeling like a kid on Christmas morning.

It only took two weeks to get in for a consultation with the new ob-gyn. It was the most hopeful I had felt in a long time. The paper that wrapped the patient chair had no chance with me sitting on top of it. I was so antsy, moving back and forth, that it ripped and fell off before I could even process what had happened. I was giggling at how ridiculous I would probably look when the doctor walked in. Torn paper, sweaty palms, and a nervous smile. Who in their right mind would be so happy to have a surgical consultation?

He walked in, introduced himself, and went over all the risks, which of course, I was well read up on. He was going to do the surgery robotically to be less invasive, and he wanted to bring in an ob-gyn oncologist to help with the surgery. He gave me the card for the ones he would want to work with and asked that I make the appointments for a consultation with them, as well. I won't lie: I was a little disappointed to be walking out without a scheduled surgery, but I felt positive that we were heading in the right direction. Meanwhile, I called and scheduled my appointment with the hematologist, the oncologist, and a high-risk ob-gyn, for when I became pregnant.

A wonderful friend of my mom's knew a hematologist whom her family saw often and sent the information to me. I called and tried to schedule an appointment. The sweetest front-desk lady answered, and it turned out, I needed to get my blood results from the fertility doctor emailed over to them so the doctor could go over the results to decide if I needed an appointment. So again, I was told to wait. I'd like to consider myself a pretty patient person, but the days had become long and the wait, irritating.

A little time had passed and the same sweet lady called and made my appointment. The doctor was incredible; I left crying that day I first saw him. Tears of joy that he didn't think I was a complete loon for wanting one more baby after all the complications. He listened to me; he cared about how he could help, and I felt completely full of love. If anything, this man was going to try to figure as much out as he could for me. And that meant the world to me. I was tired of people laughing at us and our determination to add one more to our bunch. He made me feel validated and to this day, I'm grateful for him and his entire staff. He went over my health history and labs extensively and took blood while I was there. I received my lab results back and made a follow-up appointment. I was going to have to take baby aspirin while trying to conceive and once we got pregnant, I'd add Lovenox shots to the mix. He again assured me that once we were pregnant, he would be watching very closely and that I was important to him and to my family, so he would take great care of me. It's hard to find doctors like that these days, but there he was.

The next week, I had my high-risk ob-gyn appointment. It was in my hometown, close to our house. I knew it would be a hard appointment, but I was ready to tackle it. The doctor was very kind but also very concerned. He had gotten my images from the fertility doctor and my lab results from my appointments the week prior. He went over all my risks, and there were a lot of them. Just it being my sixth C-section presented risks. He was drawing pictures of all the horrible things that could go wrong. The placenta growing into the extremely scarred uterus and all of the horrible possibilities if it continued to grow into my organs and so on. Then he brought in the blood-clotting disorder I had just discovered I had. Being on blood thinners with my sixth C-section and the dehiscence I had was another cocktail for death or serious consequences for both my baby and me. I told him I was planning on having the surgery to fix the dehiscence. He warned that would create more scarring on my uterus and add more risks. It was undoubtedly an eye-opening appointment. Bless the doctor's heart; he was just trying to make sure I was informed that this could be an extremely bad situation.

Nothing fazed me, though—not for one second. I was just there to cross my *t*s and dot my *i*s before getting pregnant. I just needed to make sure I had the doctor lined up to keep an eye out on my future baby. In hindsight, I must have come across as a real whacko. I had a big smile on my face, thanked him for his time, and went on my way. Nothing he could say would stop me from moving forward in this journey. After all, I was walking with the Lord, and He was guiding my steps once again.

I was getting pretty fed up with all the appointments. I found myself at a new doctor's office almost weekly. Some days, I was discouraged and just over having to deal with it all. But my husband and I would just keep trudging forward, even when we felt like we were flat stuck in the mud. Thank the Lord, He understands how human we can be at times.

Again, I found myself in a waiting room. This time, I was at the oncologist gynecologist. I was called back quickly and found myself twitching on chair paper again. The sound of the crinkling under me, the tapping of my fingers beside me, and my heartbeat felt like a train running ten minutes late for its next stop. I was tired of this situation, of these emotions, and especially of the insecurities. The doctor walked in, and I put on my big fake smile, hoping it would end soon. He agreed to be a part of my surgical team. They wanted him because he was used to weird and complicated surgeries, being in the cancer field. Before I left, he asked if I could schedule an MRI and follow-up appointment with him after I get that done.

Argh! Another dang appointment and another stinking test. None of these appointments were close to home, except the high-risk ob-gyn's office. So with my fake smile still plastered on my face, I agreed and waited until he left the room to allow a tear to fall down my tired and sore eyes and onto that crinkly paper.

I like to talk to God throughout my day. It gives me comfort, and I love having a genuine relationship with Him. I told Him I was weary. This was all getting to be a little much. I had kids at home with crazy schedules that I had to keep up with, and I worked part-time at a gym. With every appointment I booked, I had to ask a family member to watch my two youngest, so I could really concentrate on getting everything out of the appointments I could. I was tired of leaving my girls, I was tired of getting my shifts covered, and most of all, I was just plain tired—more so mentally and emotionally than physically. I was like a crazy train with no breaks, an emotional roller-coaster with attitude ups and downs. I can't say it enough: I am so thankful for God's grace and mercy. Some days, I'd be feeling high on the unwavering peace that passes no understanding, and other days, I was knee-deep in sorrow and pity parties. I pulled myself together and walked to the front of the office and made my follow-up and my MRI test appointments.

The MRI was a quick schedule, and I was thankful for that. Again, I found myself at the oncologist on that nasty crinkly paper. I wasn't nervous this time. I just wanted it to be over. I was ready to schedule my surgery and get the ball rolling. The doc came in with a big smile on his face. "Well you're good to go!"

He saw the perplexed look on my face and let out a chuckle. He pulled up his laptop with the images of the MRI; it was normal aside from the old C-section scar. He then asked when I was planning on trying to conceive since it was clear. *Is this for real?*

He explained he wasn't sure what had happened between the time I had the HSG and the MRI, but everything looked good. Of course, for months I had prayed for some sort of miracle or a sign that I was doing the right thing. Even though I had prayed and believed in our plans, I was still shocked when we received the miracle. The images from the original HSG terrified every doctor we had brought it to. Now, we were healed from the only thing that had stopped us from moving forward. I ran out of the office to call my husband.

He kept asking me to repeat myself, and even once he heard what I was saying, he didn't believe his ears. We were both overjoyed with the news. God granted us peace and had performed a miracle; we knew for sure we were on the right path.

A few months had passed, and I started taking hormone pills after every ovulation and an aspirin every night. Every year in December, we'd go to San Francisco to celebrate the birth of my favorite person in the world, my husband Jordan. Before we knew it, we were on the plane, headed for a weekend of fun and excitement. Little did we know, it would be our most memorable trip to date. It had been a few months of trying with no luck, so I figured it wasn't going to happen again. I brought a few tests, just in case, because I wanted to know the very moment it happened.

We enjoyed our first day in California as we always do, going to our favorite spots. We planned a wine tasting in Napa Valley for the second day. It was still pretty early to find out, but I decided to take a test anyway. Much to my surprise, it was positive! Two little pink lines stared right in my face! Instant joy and terror hit again. Needless to say, I had the best sober wine tasting ever! I booked an appointment with my hematologist and ob-gyn for soon after we'd arrive home.

After my appointments, I started my Lovenox shots. I had a cocktail of Lovenox shots, progesterone pills, aspirin, and prenatal vitamins every day, alongside lots of prayers. We tried not to get excited; we had let ourselves do so in the past, and it made the losses sting. Who were we kidding, though—we were through the moon!

Those first few weeks seemed like torture. Trying to be sane and let the past not affect us was more challenging than we expected. I dreaded my first appointment and the days that lead up to it. Every little loss of symptom sent me into a panic. I had a heart monitor and loved watching my resting heartbeat rise every day, just like it was supposed to—due to the increase of hormones in my body.

One night, six weeks into my pregnancy, I noticed my resting heart rate had dropped four beats per minute. I just knew it was over, I ripped the watch off of my wrist, and threw it across the room where it shattered alongside my heart. Jordan comforted me and told me I was looking for things to worry about, but I saw through his beautiful green eyes; he was sad, too. I mourned what I thought was the loss of another sweet baby. I felt lifeless once again. I didn't bother making an appointment for the next day; I figured if I made it to my eight-week appointment, we would deal with things then.

The office called and booked me at seven weeks instead of eight, and we went in like a ball of nerves, fearful but with a smidge of hope burning inside. And there it was, the most beautiful thing we had ever seen . . . 180 beats per minute. Our tiny miracle was there with his little heart thumping away. We had made it through our first milestone. A small measure of our nerves were settled, but we had a long way to go.

At ten weeks I found myself lying on the floor in a puddle of tears, calling Jordan who at the time, was out of town. Previously, at the eight week mark, we were able to hear a strong heartbeat through our at home Doppler. But I couldn't find the heartbeat. The only thing I heard was silence through my hour-long, desperate search. Again, he put on his brave voice for me, telling me it was going to be okay, even when I was hysterically crying, thinking we had lost another one. I knew he was shaken though. He was right. Everything turned out fine.

I mourned the loss of our baby several more times, and each time, I was proven wrong. I went for a walk with my sweet and dear friend Niki and our youngest kids one day. She gave me a present, something I cherished dearly. It was a necklace with a mustard seed, and it said, "All things are possible." What a wonderful daily reminder. I put it on and didn't take it off after that day.

At twenty weeks, we felt such a huge relief. We were still going to the high-risk doctors, and they performed ultrasounds every month. Everything had been progressing beautifully. My placenta was over my cervix, so we had to continue monthly ultrasounds, even though I would have a repeat C-section anyway. We loved the opportunity to see our precious baby every month.

It was such a wonderful time of year. Our oldest was playing baseball, my husband was coaching, and the kids would be out of school soon. I looked forward to summer every year; I'm one of those crazy moms who are sad when the kids go back to school. We were kicking off the beginning of summer and my twenty-seventh week of pregnancy by going to a baseball tournament. We stayed in a hotel, enjoyed time with our baseball family, and breathed easy with baby "Judah," growing strong and me feeling great.

We got back to town with a full car of dirty clothes, tired kids, and happy hearts. I had a routine ultrasound that morning, and we were looking forward to seeing our sweet boy. A few times, I had pain that put my body into a panic, and one time I actually passed out. Each time, I became drenched in sweat. I figured the episodes were so few and far between, and I had a lot of scarring that it must just be normal. I have a really high pain tolerance, and it really didn't bother me each time I underwent the Doppler, and Judah's heart was beating beautifully.

The ultrasound tech called us back, and she started the ultrasound. Jordan left after the ultrasound before the doc came back to take our daughter Gigi to gymnastics. He made sure to tell me to talk to the doc about the pains I had experienced a few times. With a roll of my eyes, I said, "OK, I will." He proceeded to make me promise I would say something because he knows me well enough!

So the doctor came in said the baby looked fantastic. Reluctantly, I told him about the pains. He said he wanted to take a closer look and hooked me back up to the ultrasound machine. I was watching his face as he peered at everything. Then, shock spread across his face. I grasped my necklace and started talking to God like I always had when doubt and fear crept in during my pregnancy.

He pointed and outlined my uterus until we got to the bottom left part, where my bladder was located. He asked if I saw it, but there was nothing there. He called in the ultrasound tech to show her, and they were both dumbfounded. He asked me to wait in a conference room while he called a few other ob-gyns who were located in the hospital. I could feel the blood leave my face and my heart start to pound through my chest while trying to keep a cool face. I texted Jordan just to give him a heads up that the doctors where conferencing on how to handle the situation, and that at the moment, I wasn't really sure what was going on. After a bit the doctors came in and sat me down. Again, I was holding strong to that mustard seed necklace and the promise I know the Lord was fulfilling.

The great news was that Judah looked perfect, an instant relief for me. The bad news was that they couldn't see if there was any uterus lining at all on the bottom, and my bladder was plastered to it. If Judah kicked too hard, or if I had a strong contraction, he could be sent straight through my bladder causing me to bleed to death within minutes— and likely he would pass in a few minutes, as well. Being on blood thinners made this all the riskier. I was almost twenty-eight weeks; babies born at twenty-eight weeks had a high survival rate. Again, the blood left my face and I put on an autopilot smile, my go-to face when I don't know how else to react.

The medical team made a plan for me to stay at the university hospital where they had special surgeons for both my C-section and for my bladder. I was instructed to go home, pack, and head straight there. I didn't think about what would have happened if my husband hadn't made me tell the doctors about the pain that day. It wouldn't have been found unless they were looking for something off, and it was very off.

I got home and met Jordan and our two youngest. I started doing laundry and picking up from our weekend. My parents came in the house to take the girls for us and then pick up the big kids from school. They were all telling me to stop cleaning and get packed to go. How could I go! I wasn't ready! I was in denial. This baby needed to cook some more in the safety of my body, and I needed to take care of my family before I could go anywhere. I had just started setting up the nursery; it was mid-baseball season, and I had so many fun summer plans for our kids. My brain was checked out of reality.

I packed my bags and we got in the car. It was one of those feelings, like life was happening around you but you are in slow-motion, watching it happen.

We arrived at the hospital, and I was still in denial. I checked in and was sent to my room, Room 405. The nurse came in and went over my health history and had me change into a hospital gown. The doctors had ordered a steroid shot to help develop Judah's lungs. The doctors came in soon after and started to go over everything. I grasped my mustard seed, trying to process what was going on. She seemed pretty certain we would be delivering in a few days and scheduled the urologist surgeons, the NICU staff, the anesthesiologist, the blood bank, and an oncologist since they deal with weird surgeries to all come in and talk to us that evening. We were on information overload, and I sat with the necklace in my grasp and my goofy don't-know-how-to-react smile plastered on my face the entire time.

All of the doctors commented on how calm and collective I appeared. If only they knew the rip tides of emotions that were tearing me from limb to limb on the inside. I tried to take my mind away from all the worst-case scenarios they were obligated to inform me of. The bladder reconstruction, hysterectomy, blood transfusion, baby risks with being born so early—all too much to process. From finally feeling confident in my pregnancy to having the floor ripped out from underneath me.

That night, sleep was impossible; my mind was all over the place. The next day, they came in for baby monitoring, and there he was, with his beautiful baby heart pumping away. Happy tears soaked my face; he was inside, happy as can be and loving every second of the life God was blessing him with. We are all on God's timing. I felt peace fall over me once again—it was time to put on my battle helmet and get ready for a bumpy ride. God had me and, most importantly, God had our precious baby boy, and I was going to love him every second I could. We don't know God's plans and having to trust in them can be almost impossible some days. I love every single baby who didn't make it here on earth, and I look forward to holding every one for an eternity one day. Nothing will ever take away the pain of losing them, and nothing will help me understand why it happened to them. But I will trust in God, and I can find comfort in knowing I will hold them one day. Praising God in the storms is so difficult, but it is necessary for healing. I was in a place of fully relying on God.

The next day came and went, and I felt great. They switched from my Lovenox shots once a day to Heparin twice a day in case of an emergency surgery. They could correct the effects of Heparin easier than Lovenox. Judah sounded fantastic once again on the monitor. The doctors said they were going to have a meeting with all the head high-risk ob-gyns at the hospital and at the practice to see how long they would let me try to grow him inside. They had to weigh all the risks and come up with a best-case plan. They put a thick IV into my arm so at any moment, they could rush me into surgery and give me a blood transfusion. It's a weird feeling to have my body feeling so great and healthy, but in reality, be a ticking time bomb.

The first day, they said I could take a wheelchair outside to get some fresh air. Then, they let me go out walking, as long as my husband was with me, and I didn't go too far. Before we knew it, a whole week had passed, and everything was going as well as it could go. Originally, they said I would deliver in days. Then, they decided I should try to hold off until thirty-two weeks. After talking with them and saying I felt great for the most part (I had a few episodes of pain that had faded away), they decided to set the surgery date for the thirty-six-week mark.

I was excited to get to that day. At thirty-six weeks, the baby would have only minimal NICU time, if any at all. It was daunting to think I'd be at the hospital for eight weeks on bed rest, but I knew it was for our baby boy. The hardest part was not having my five other precious kids with me. I love taking care of them and seeing their sweet faces every day.

Our family and friends stepped up and took care of us. It was such an outpouring of love. The days moved slowly, and I looked forward to visits from friends and family, especially those precious five kiddos. My husband spent every night with me. I tried to hide how bad I needed him there with me, but it didn't matter; he knew I did. He brought in a big-screen monitor and set up Netflix, brought me fun food, and went on daily walks with me. I don't know what I would have done without him there for my sanity. The staff at the hospital were incredible, always smiling and positive. Even in the midst of that chaos, God was orchestrating even the little things. The sweetest lady came in every day to mop the floors and would put her hands up and say a quick prayer. Judah was surrounded by God's love. Every week that passed, I celebrated that he was growing stronger and would have to fight less on the outside. There was nothing more motivating than knowing every day you were able to hold on, your child grew stronger.

Pretty soon Father's Day arrived, and I was thirty weeks pregnant. The thirty-week mark made me confident that we would make it to that thirty-six-week mark. I woke up with some pain and figured it would just go away. I planned for my husband to pick up the kids from my parents house and take them to a movie and lunch. After all, he deserved a fun day and some fresh air! I didn't mention how bad the pain was getting because I was in denial that anything could or would happen that day. I never really complained and tried to stay as positive as I could. So when I mentioned I wasn't feeling so hot and had some lower left side pain, they started preparing for anything. I was a "hard stick" as they called it, and it usually took a few times before the IV would work. So they sent in the big guns to use an ultrasound to get it in quickly as they pumped fluids in my other IV site. The doctors came in and ordered an ultrasound and hooked me up to the monitors. I was having contractions and Judah didn't like them. I called Jordan and told him it was probably nothing but maybe he should turn around, or I could keep him posted. I've never gone into labor at thirty weeks; it was most likely dehydration, and they were giving me fluids. The ultrasound came back that my bladder didn't look great from the contractions, and Judah's heart was decelerating. They gave me another shot for his lungs. Jordan walked in, and I heard the doctor tell him, "It's go time."

"What? No, I'm sorry, but I'm waiting until thirty-six weeks. You just tell that baby and my body to slow down!"

About that time, the blood work came back that the Heparin had worn off, and I'd be able to stay awake during surgery. They pumped me full of magnesium to help with the risk of preemie brain bleeds . . . not something I wanted to hear before my tiny baby was about to be born. As soon as the magnesium hit, the room spun, and I was soaked in sweat. At that same time, my precious kiddos and parents walked in. I tried to hold it together, pretend I was feeling okay. It was tough for a good fifteen minutes, and then the magnesium was tolerable. They wheeled me back and told Jordan to wait—they would come get him later. This was a huge miracle for us. Every case scenario they had given us outlined he wouldn't be able to go back with me. Even if we had made it to the planned operation at thirty-six weeks, we weren't expecting him to be allowed in surgery. But on that day, things went differently. I was more than relieved that he would be by my side. The anesthesiologist was putting my back block in when my blood pressure tanked, and the nurse held on to me. Once again, my body was drenched in sweat. They laid me down and gave me a minute to compose myself.

Surgery started and I prayed like never before. They pulled Judah out, and I heard gasps and a lot of "oh my goshes" around the room. They took down the drape that was separating me from my baby, and I saw his sweet, little face for the first time. They showed me his cord that had what they called a true knot. Sometimes, babies are born with knots in their cords, but a true knot is one so tight that it loses circulation. It's rare. The cord was also squeezing his neck, wrapped around it twice. Every contraction I had experienced had pulled it tighter. His life was flashing before his eyes, and we had no idea.

And I had been trying to stop his delivery from happening that day! The doctors prepared us that it's normal to not hear a baby born that early cry. When Judah let out a mighty cry, Jordan and I lost it. Tears and grins from ears to ears. Again, God was comforting us. There was a whole NICU staff in the room, and they took Judah once he was born.

I was so nervous to learn how big he was. My other five kids where born small at full term. My biggest was six pounds, seven ounces, and my smallest was five pounds, ten ounces. Being ten weeks early, I dreaded hearing the number. They got excited when they announced he was three pounds, eleven ounces and seventeen inches long! Wow! Another huge miracle. God was just showing off at this point. I love it when God comes in and makes it blatantly obvious His Wonder and Majesty are at work. When the NICU staff had prepared us previously, they said to not freak out when they put him inside a plastic bag. They do that to help him keep heat. They were all laughing when Judah wasn't fully fitting into the bag and called him the "Big Thirty-Weeker." Jordan went to be with Judah while they got him stable.

My surgery was going better than they could have expected. It took longer than my other surgeries because they were repairing a lot of things, but in the end, I didn't need a blood transfusion, which shocked all the doctors. They put Judah in a little crib to transport him to the NICU, and they stopped by my head for me to talk to him for a second. I told him happy birthday and how much I loved him and how very proud I was of him. In return, he let out another big cry and turned his head to me. That was the best feeling in the world. I had been told all along I would be put under for surgery and not be able to meet my son until I woke up. Yet, there I was, talking to my precious miracle, and he answered back. You can't tell me this wasn't God's work.

After the repairs, they sewed me back up, and I couldn't get wheeled out of there fast enough. I passed good old #405 on my way to recovery, and all of my family and Jordan's family were waiting in that room, waving to me as I passed by. I still remember seeing my dad's face and the relief he had in his eyes. They joined me soon after, in recovery. The nurse I had that day was the same sweet nurse who had checked us in. I hadn't seen her since. It had come full-circle; she had us again. She really fought for me to go see Judah right away. As soon as the NICU had Judah settled and on oxygen, she wheeled me back in my hospital bed to see him. I still didn't have any feeling in my legs, yet. There he was—all three pounds and eleven ounces of pure miracle perfection. I was able to put my hand in the hole of his glass box, and he held onto my finger. My husband had officially gotten the best Father's Day present known to man. His precious baby boy was safe; his wife was safe, and God had us all in the palm of His Hand. Before they wheeled me back so they could run some tests, I reached down and grabbed my necklace—all things are possible—and put it on his enclosed crib. The necklace was in his room until the day we were discharged. God's timing was perfect. Had Judah not been born that day, the outcome would have been tragic. Later, we found out the cord was inserted in the side of the placenta, and my placenta had been failing, as well. It was small and losing its life. How in the world did all that factoring in create such a big baby, born ten weeks early? I'll tell you how . . . God.

The NICU stay was an incredibly difficult situation. I was discharged five days after my C-section. They didn't warn me how hard it was going to be to leave my precious baby behind and go home with empty arms. Pumping every three hours produced a lonely feeling. I'll never forget the agony of driving away and leaving my baby in someone else's care. I won't lie: I fell apart. I know God was in control; after all, He had given us all these incredible miracles! But between the sadness of not having my baby to hold, the hormones raging through my body, and no sleep, I was a mess. Just like losing a baby, you don't fully understand the pain until having to go through it. I found myself realizing how painful it was to have a NICU baby. The staff Judah had was a group of complete angels on earth.

There were so many highs and lows. We would take one step forward than take giant steps backward. The first time I got to hold him, I melted into my seat. It was an out-of-this-world experience to finally hold that baby. He beat all the odds on several occasions from the moment of his conception to that day. He tested positive for a rare disease, but after several tests, it was finally ruled out. They thought he had a brain bleed, but it turned out to be a few little cysts that weren't a big deal. He had what the NICU refers to as Brady's, which all preemies get. Brady's are when the babies' heart rates drop extremely low. One day he experienced back-to-back-to-back ones, and they thought maybe he was sick. Sometimes, the infants can pull it back up themselves; other times, nurses have to give them some help. The alarms sent chills down my spine. They would go off when the heart rate was low, and I would panic. It turned out, he wasn't sick though. The feeding tube was too short since he grew so fast. They lowered it, and he felt much better.

He was packing on weight daily. He had a really hard time learning to eat, and that's what slowed us down the most. I was getting nervous because my big kids starting school in eleven days, and he still wasn't eating like he should be to go home. The hospital was forty-five minutes away from our house, and our kids went to three different schools with three different drop off and pick up times. That meant, I'd have hardly any time to be at the hospital with Judah. I kept praying that we would have one last miracle and get him home.

I fell apart one day when the nurse said there was no way he would be ready to go home by the time school started. I shut the curtain of his tiny room and just cried my eyes out. I told the Lord how thankful I was for our miracle and that I was ashamed to be anything but grateful. I needed that peace again; after all, I'm human. God moved mountains, and the necklace with "all things are possible" was proven faithful once again. It turned out Judah was anemic, and he was so tired, he couldn't stay awake to eat. As soon as they gave him shots to help, he was eating like a champ. They called to schedule our discharge class, and I screamed with excitement on the phone. That was the final step for our baby boy, the one we had waited for, for years, through tears and fears and faith—to be going home! Wouldn't you know it, God was showing off again . . . our baby boy came home one day before school started.

That day was a huge day for us. I had the kids all dressed in matching shirts; we got doughnuts and gifts for the staff; and we headed in with our huge family full of smiles. For some reason, it was taking a little longer to discharge. Let's be real—that reason was God. Our kids went to the playroom to hang out while we waited with Judah.

Our hospital room neighbor was another miracle baby. A firecracker born on the 4th of July at just one pound. I had met her mom while in the hospital when we were both on the pregnant side of things. She was such a sweetheart. Her water had broken at seventeen weeks, and she managed to stay pregnant with no infection until around twenty-seven weeks. The baby was a fighter; she kept defying all odds. Some days, while I was rocking Judah, I could hear her mama crying. It was hard to hear another mom suffering with fear for her child's life. I would pray over them every day from our little corner. The day baby Judah was being discharged, I heard the nurses in a panic. Judah's precious little neighbor wasn't sounding good— something was wrong. Immediately, I lifted my hands toward her room and went into a deep prayer with the Lord.

"Please Lord, be with this precious baby girl. Give the doctors wisdom and guide their hands in helping her."

I could feel the power of the Holy Spirit that day. I experienced goosebumps while praying. I looked over and saw that necklace dangling in Judah's room.

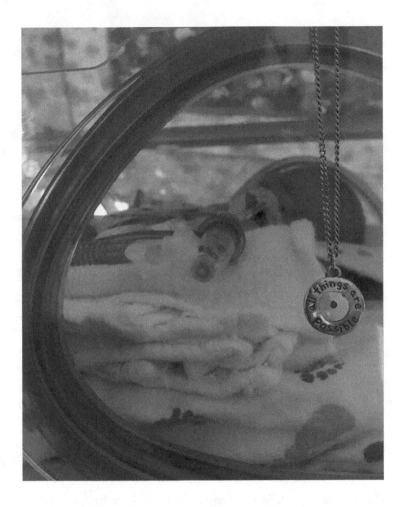

I knew it was time to pass it on. I slipped in and put it on our NICU neighbor's breast pump, and we left the NICU. What a glorious day that was. After a total of seventy-six days between me then him staying in the hospital, we were headed home with our miracle baby.

A few days later, I got a text from the mom of that precious baby. She told me how much the necklace meant and that the day she got it turned out to be perfect timing. Her baby had been super sick, and she had been more than worried. God had performed a huge miracle, though, and her baby was recovering with the help of her medicine. The day of her text, she was doing fantastic, and I hoped that her incredible story gets told one day.

There were days I truly had faith the size of a mustard seed; other days I had faith the size of a mountain. God was with us each and every day, regardless of what size faith we could muster up. He was with each and every passing tear. He doesn't promise us an easy life, but he promises a faithful one. I pray that mustard seed travels far and wide and encourages many more to come. God's timing is perfect and our precious Judah is proof.

****

After reading every journey, tears slip down my face to form a giant puddle of compassion and love for our sisters and their families. Judah is indeed like a bright and beautiful rainbow after the storm; he is a reminder of God's faithfulness to us all. A beautiful fairytale ending written by God himself; although, as Katie said, their journey to Judah was not easy, but they never gave up, remaining faithful. I asked Katie if I could share a beautiful poem she wrote after one of their losses. I believe it will warm and comfort your heart.

Here I am again with a broken heart,
No life left inside I didn't want you to part,
Those two little lines made me love you so much,
Now I'll never get the chance to give you the motherly touch,
Tears streaming down I've been here before,
I had so many plans for you and your siblings in store,
Now your up in heaven with my other babies I love,
I have to wait here on earth until I hold you all above,
This isn't fair and it makes me so sad,
We never got the chance to be your mom and your dad,
We will love you from here until we hold you one day,
I hope you know the deep love I have for you I pray,
Jesus please hold my babies for me,
And help mend my broken heart,
Until their beautiful faces I see
During my heavenly start.
Until then give me peace I pray,
For in my deepest sorrow I still praise you on this day.

Wow, chills again. When I close my eyes, I can imagine Jesus holding each and every baby we've all lost, loving on them in only the way He can. It takes a deep faith and a distinctive piece of our soul to praise Him in our deepest sorrows. Such a difficult thing, but when we do,

He strengthens us and becomes our peace and calm. I say, "Amen" to Katie's prayer . . . Amen, Lord, please heal every broken heart.

Thank you for sharing your beautiful heart and poem, Katie. You are a true inspiration to us all!

Life is a series of miracles, tiny and vast. I see them and feel them every day. They are all around us, exquisite and powerful. Look for them. Never forget you can be the answer to someone else's prayer. Sisterhood, while necklaces are circulating all around the world, so are tiny seeds of faith, hope, and living, breathing miracles. It makes my heart and soul sing!

I have had the immense privilege of sharing in friendship and ministry with a woman who has truly been the hands and feet of Jesus. When I shared a necklace with her, I prayed specifically that God would give her the desires of her heart and that she would reap the harvest of the generous seeds she had planted. Renee is a woman who always says "yes" when someone is in need. She is there, time and time again, with a helpful hand.

She has worked hard to get where she is in life, so she will be the first one to encourage you to do the same. She has given so many a hand-up, not a handout. I cannot count the times Renee has asked me (and many others) to share anonymous financial gifts with those in need. She has helped multiple families follow their dreams of having children. When hefty bills stood in front of dreams, she was there to knock them down.

This is one of the many reasons why I wanted to share a necklace with Renee. I know she has accomplished many goals and followed her own dreams; however, there are still some she is waiting to come to fruition. Although she would like to marry and have children, this has not stopped her for praying and helping others do the same. Talk about selfless! Helping others have what your own heart desires.

There is so much to learn from people like her who give back before they even receive. Never give up on your dreams; never put God in a box. He is the One whom left Heaven for us; surely there is nothing too big for Him. He is infinite in strength, and I know he wants Renee to have the desires of her heart.

Psalm 20:4 (NLT): "May He grant your hearts desires and make all your plans succeed."

This is Renee's story.

7

Meet Renee

Trailblazer

My name is Renee, and I am blessed that I have friendships and many interactions with most of the women in this book. Like the other women who have shared their stories, I have had my own struggles and doubts in many areas of my life. I have conquered some and still struggle with others, even to this day. I hope my story inspires you to continue forward, whatever your journey is, and to never give up, no matter what the struggles are or how difficult they may be. The most important strategies are to support each other, have a plan, and learn who you are and what your purpose is. Remember, it's your own journey; try not to compare yours to someone else's. We are not the Robinsons or the Joneses. We don't need to be what other people are or worry about what they have. We are unique to God and have our own role to play in His design. We need to remind ourselves of this, and sometimes, we need reminding from others around us.

One of my first struggles was my having bowed legs. As a young child, toddler age, I was diagnosed with Rickets. Rickets disease is a problem that is often found in young children, and it can cause deformity and fractures of the bones. The doctors decided to place my legs in casts for a time to see if they would grow straight. Well, I can tell you my legs are still bowed to this day, but that has not stopped me from swimming, running, playing volleyball, or doing all the other things kids did and adults do.

I am short, so as a child, I felt like I stuck out, or more like, wasn't seen. The other kids would make comments like, "Man, are you short!" or even ask me if I was a midget. I remember thinking they must believe I can't do the same things they can do. I assumed they thought I was helpless, but that was far from the case. There were a number of times I would run and swim longer than the other kids and even scored well on the Presidential Physical Fitness Test we had to do each year. As a young child, around seven or eight years old, my dad taught me how to play volleyball. This meant I had to learn how to serve the ball behind the line and get it over the net to the other team. No serving mid-court because I was a young kid.

I practiced, and at one point, I was able to serve the volleyball to anywhere on the other side of the net. So eventually, I would only play with the adults. My parents asked me at one point if my small size bothered me, and I stated that it did. After that conversation, at about age twelve or thirteen, my parents sent me to Johns Hopkins University to find out if they could help with my small size. Sadly, they informed us there was nothing they could do. I would have loved my legs to be longer and straighter, but that was never going to happen. The doctors told me that people who had my condition would most likely need knee replacements later in life. I still walk fast, get around well, and have no complaints with my physical disabilities.

The second struggle I faced was also as a young child. On the last day of third grade, walking home from school after a discussion with my teacher where she said she would need to talk with my parents, I was upset. I didn't understand why she needed to talk with my parents or what I had done wrong. I would find out later that I had a learning disability that soon would be diagnosed as dyslexia. I had to be sent to another school, so I could attend special education classes for my learning disability. I literally had to ride the "short bus" at times to and from school. I remember going to special education classes and feeling stupid and inadequate. I had trouble with spelling and writing and sometimes reading. I felt like I was not as smart as the rest of the kids. I remember getting book reports back with all kinds of red marks on them. I remember feeling like no matter what I did, my writing and spelling were never going to be good enough.

This feeling followed me for the rest of my school years. I knew I had trouble with spelling and writing, but I didn't feel I deserved to be treated like I was not as smart as the rest of the kids in class, let alone being placed in a class for kids with learning difficulties. I felt like I was being separated from what society perceived as the "smart kids." The skills that helped me during my school years were my memory and reading comprehension. Those were my two strongest abilities, and they aided me considerably. I know without a doubt that without my strength in those two abilities, I wouldn't have made it through school.

To this day, there are times when I get irritated with people who correct my spelling or writing. They have no idea what it took for me to get to this point with my writing. I thank God for spell check! I now have a Master's Degree in nursing, which involved a lot of writing in each class. I completed my master's with a lot more time and effort than those who were much better writers than I. I know I had to take more time and energy to complete those class papers, so I scheduled time accordingly. To this day, when I write a paper or a long document, I have someone else look it over for me. I remember a conversation with my mom when I told her I was going to get my Master's Degree. She simply stated, "I know you will finish it because you always finish what you start."

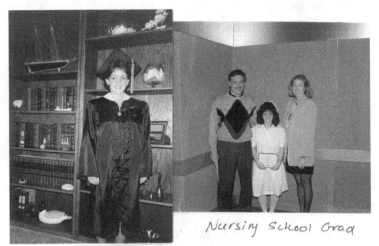

High School Grad

Nursing School Grad

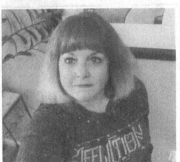

me Now Master's and all. ☺

Another struggle surfaced when I was about eight years old. This struggle would be my parents' separation and eventual divorce. I remember the day my parents told my brother and me they weren't going to be together any-more. They invited us into the family room. My brother and I sat on the couch as they dropped the bomb that they weren't going to be together anymore. I ran up to my room and cried. It was such a shock. I hadn't seen it coming. I thought, "What is going to happen to us and what caused this?" These were just a few of the things going through my mind at that time. Back then, divorce was uncommon and considered a taboo. I wondered what my friends and others would think.

This was just one other thing to deal with besides my dyslexia, short stature, and bowed legs. What a piece of work I was! What a mess! Looking back, I should have gone to counseling to deal with all of the negative feel-ings I harbored. I dealt with feelings of anger, inadequacy, and at times, I acted like I had a chip on my shoulder. I felt the experience of my parents' divorce was molding my thoughts about parenting and relationships. If they couldn't stay together and make it work and have love, what chance did I have? I told myself I would not let a child go through that. I remember talking with my moth-er on the phone many years after their divorce, and she said she felt like she was the reason I was still alone and not married. I responded that it was more complicated than that. I feel like relationships are complicated and can't be solved like math problems, or even be rationalized out . . . and why should they be?

We all have challenges. Most of us know what those challenges are and don't need or like to be reminded of them. As an adult, my challenge has been finding the right person for me to marry. Sadly, this battle continues to this day. I've always known I want to be married and have children, but I also want to have a loving, supportive relationship and am not willing to go through the type of relationship my parents had, which ended in divorce. In the Bible, Genesis 2:18 discusses how it was "not good" for the man to be alone but together, Adam and Eve were something far stronger and more magnificent than either of them could have been alone. Alone we are just parts of a whole.

Throughout the years, I have seen some of my women friends have children with no support from the child's other parent. I have also seen women get married and then ultimately, get divorced. I never want to be in that situation or put a child through that trauma. I would rather have no children than to put a child through that. I know what it's like. I want my child to know a loving, kind relationship and not experience what I saw with my parents' poor relationship. In my mind, there are enough children in poverty, parentless and hungry, and I refuse to add to this dilemma in our society. I know what divorce feels like from a child's perspective, and I want my child to be protected from those same struggles. I think every parent wants their child to have a better life than they had. I don't believe that having a child because an individual wants to be a parent or not considering the consequences of sexual intimacy is selfish, but I believe life is more than just about me. I feel whatever I do and say causes a ripple effect. The ripple effect can have either good or bad consequences.

The ripple effect is one's actions, seen or unseen, which affect others, even though the individual may not see or understand the unforeseen consequences of those words or actions. There is a tendency to believe that at times, our actions only affect us. This couldn't be further from the truth. I want to have a positive effect on those around me, in all of society. I want to see the bigger picture and have a vision that extends beyond myself. I am talking about community and working with one another to make each other a better, stronger version of ourselves.

The Bible talks about community in Hebrews 10:24–25 (NIV): "Let us consider how we may spur one another on toward love and good deeds, not giving up meeting together, as some are in the habit of doing, but encouraging one another—and all the more—as you see the Day approaching." It is not uncommon to shut yourself in, not want to go out, and avoid interaction with others when feeling down and have nothing to contribute or are going through a difficult period in life. This is the most important time to be with friends and family, let them lend support, and be part of a community. In turn, you do the same for them in their times of need.

The community, good friends, and family have helped me in difficult times. It's important to be there for others in their times of need. There are so many ways to be of help to the people around you and even those who are strangers. You never know how lending a hand to a stranger can impact their lives, maybe even set them on a path to pay it forward to some else. It is wonderful to contribute to the concept of paying it forward. Remember, someone at some point may have given you an opportunity you didn't realize at the time, and you may not have deserved or expected it.

What about one's faith? How does this affect our journeys? How hard would our journey be with little or no faith? You may experience that feeling of hopelessness or feeling like there is nothing that can be done to change your circumstances. I remember watching TV after the Tsunami hit Indonesia and parts of India several years ago,and how devastating it was for those people. All the outpouring of support to those people in need, during their time of crisis, was wonderful to see. What struck me was during one of the interviews, a woman in one of the affected areas was asked how she felt about all the support she and many others received during this devastating time. She responded by saying she had no idea anyone cared. I couldn't fathom anyone feeling this way, but sadly, I've learned many people feel like this. They feel like no one cares, or they have no hope. They have little or no faith in themselves, others, or even a higher power, whomever that may be for them. I know faith has also helped me during difficult times, especially in the last ten years of my journey. I say the last ten years because that is the time I really started to understand faith.

Going to church and meeting with my church family, who have helped changed my life—and continue to do so to this day—is how my faith continues to grow. It has also helped me really understand the importance of community and helping others. I was so grateful to be part of their lives and some of the stories told by the women in this book. I thank God, I am able to help others in any way I can. The Bible asks us, "Do to others as you would have them do to you." (Luke 6:31, NIV) Mathew 25:40 reads, "Most certainly I tell you, in as much as you did it to one of the least of these my *brothers,* you did it to me." These are just a few of the concepts I try to live by, exemplify, or as we say at church, "reverberate."

I remember watching one of Craig Groeschel's sermons and he said, "Everyone gets someplace but very few people get there on purpose."

"How prophetic" I thought!

Of course, you can't get someplace without knowing where you want to go; you can't even come up with a plan of how you want to get there. In Proverbs 29:18 it shares the concept "where there is no vision, the people perish." Can you imagine having no idea about your future or purpose? How would you get through life? I suspect the answer would be *very poorly*, and without purpose or intent, I am positive our relationships with others would suffer, as well.

These ideas have stuck with me from the first time I heard them and continue to mold my actions and be in the forefront of my thinking to this day. My last thought for you would be, no matter what your struggles or hardships are, find faith, purpose, and meaning for your life with a group of people who lift you up, increase your faith, and help you on your own journey, no matter how hard it is or impossible it seems. Remember, we all have a purpose and get increased strength and faith from a loving community of friends and family.

****

When I gave Renee her necklace and eventually asked her to share her story I remember thinking to myself there are so many women I know who do not have their own children. Yet they are like a mother to many, giving advice, lending a hand (or money) but most of all, setting the example of what it means to be the hands and feet of Jesus.

Some of my friends and family have chosen not to have children, some physically cannot and others, like Renee, are still holding onto faith and hope that their dreams will still happen!

As Renee has helped many others' dreams come true in growing their families, I pray that God will bless her beyond her wildest dreams!

I thought it was important in this Sisterhood to honor all the women out there who are mothering in a different capacity. To say thank you for all that you are doing. Some days it may seem like no one notices, but we do! You are making a difference in the world, and we want to say thank you!

I love Renee's loving and motherly advice: if you feel lost along the way do not lose hope! Create a plan, cast a vision, keep the faith, and put in the work! Sisters, we can do it! Keep dreaming, keep hoping, and never give up! Join our community and let's walk through life together!

By now, you can see what I mean about being surrounded by remarkable people with captivating faith! I told you I was blessed to call them friends and now you know why, and now they are your friends, too—your sisters in faith. Their journeys are overflowing with challenges, loss, heartache, hope, miracles, and triumph! But I pray that they are constant reminders of courage and promise to all, especially the brokenhearted and those facing unimaginable circumstances. In the harshest of times, keep in mind we are here for you as a community of support; you are not alone, and we are praying for you on your journey. Just as Renee is a trailblazer for her dreams and will never give up, you can defy the odds and keep going!

I have been trying to find the appropriate way to say thank you to each of these spectacular woman for sharing their stories. However, no matter what I come up with, it seems insufficient. How do you thank someone for bearing their heart and soul to the world, especially some of the darkest times in life?

My co-writing sisters, what a gift you have shared! From the deepest part of my heart—thank you! In honor of you and the Sisterhood, we will be donating a portion of the sale of each book to support groups, ministries, and non-profits related to loss, infertility, IVF, and adoption.

Another beautiful gift to be imparted are my daddy's prayers. My father, Don, is an amazing man who puts God first in his life and leads by example. Imagine a big, strong teddy bear, always there for everyone, to pray with them, comfort them, and answer the hard questions. He is a pastor, so he has preached and taught some of the best life-changing messages you could ever hear. He has officiated many weddings and funerals, and each time, you can feel God's presence, love, and peace flow with the words from his heart. My dad is there for others when many people would run the opposite direction; he is someone you want to have a friendship with and most definitely someone you go to for advice.

Pastor Don, as he is known by many, is very humble, so he would say thank you for every compliment but ask we give all the glory to God. When I asked him if I could share some of his prayers, he said, "Absolutely, I would love that." His prayers were written and prayed with such deep faith, love, and passion from the Lord.

I am thrilled and honored to share them with each of you, and if you are not quite sure what to pray or just cannot find the words, perhaps these special prayers could be your starting place. I say special because they touch my heart so, knowing that these were some of the very same prayers prayed over many of the women and families in this book.

We pray because that is how we communicate to God. He is always listening and ready to help in a time of trouble. He is the One who can restore our souls and bring a peace that transcends all knowledge.

As you are praying, know that we are standing in agreement with you and believing for your miracle. I would ask you to imagine us sitting there with you, holding your hands.

Deuteronomy 31:6 says, "Be strong and of courage, do not fear nor be afraid of them; for the Lord your God, He is the One who goes with you. He will not leave your or forsake you."

What a calming thought to know God is always with us every step of the way, loving us and wiping away our tears.

8

Meet God, Through Pastor Don

My Daddy's Prayers

A Prayer for Patience and Hope

No matter how hard it seems, don't lose hope, keep praying, keep trusting, and keep believing. The Lord is the everlasting God, the Creator of the ends of the Earth. He will not grow tired or weary, His understanding no one can comprehend. He gives strength to the weary and increases power to the weak.

The Lord longs to be gracious to you, and He waits on high to have compassion on you. For the Lord is a God of justice, a faithful God. Blessed are all those who wait for Him; they shall not be put to shame. His victory, His favor, His love, His peace, His joy, and His companionship.

I pray as you wait on the Lord for your answer with hope that you will gain a new strength and soar on wings like eagles, you will run and not get tired, you will walk and now grow weary or faint. Wait on the Lord and be of good courage and He shall strengthen your heart.

Lord of hosts, God of Israel, the One who dwells between the cherubim, You alone made heaven and earth; You alone are God! Incline Your ear and hear the prayer of Your servant, they need Your help. Lord open Your eyes and see and answer because of Your great mercy, and come quickly to help in accordance with Your love to answer the prayer, in Jesus' name, Amen!

A Prayer for Strength

We are valuable to God, our identity is in Christ, and we are God's very own possession. We worship You today, Lord. Father You are perfect in all Your ways. We praise and adore You, knowing as we do that darkness has to give way to light and defeat has to give way to victory. Our praise is where You are pleased to dwell, You inhabit the praises of Your people. Jesus' presence, along with His effective force of power—may He give us a heavenly transfusion of strength, one that rejuvenates our faith and trust. We offer our worship as confirmation of God's power to intervene miraculously, and transport us into the realm of the supernatural where there is no sickness, no luck, and only victory over the situations in our lives. We proclaim today that the assaults of the enemy upon our peace have failed, and our heart is steadfast toward You. Father, we are strengthened when we praise You, walk with You, look to You, and expect help from You. In Jesus' name, amen.

A Prayer for Encouragement

I am the salt of the earth and the light of the world. When I speak according to the Word and the will of God, Heaven responds. All things work together for my good. When I ask, I will receive; when I knock, a door will be opened to me. (If you ask what God has promised He will do it, John 14:4.)

I am the fullness of God and filled with all knowledge, as it is given by the Holy Spirit. In Him I have been given all things and enriched in every way. The truth has set me free. I am comforted by God, so I can comfort others. I am protected by God. I am healed by the stripes of Jesus. He has anointed me and put His seal of ownership on me. I am the sweet aroma of the knowledge of Christ. I am the fragrance of Christ to God, among both the saved and the lost. I am a minister of the new covenant of the Spirit of Life. Where the Spirit of Lord is, there is freedom. I am being transformed into the likeness of the Lord, ever increasing with glory from God. I have received mercy, so I will not lose heart. My inner (wo)man is being renewed day by day. I am an ambassador of Christ, and I have grace from God, so I can abound in every good work in Jesus' name, amen.

I will be confident that He who has begun a good work in me will perfect it until the day of Christ Jesus. In Jesus' name, amen.

A Prayer for a Healthy Pregnancy

I commit (insert child's name), this unborn child to You. We stand in faith during this pregnancy and birth, not giving into any fear, but possessing power, love, and a sound mind. As Your Word promises in 2 Timothy 1:7, Heavenly Father, we confess You are our refuge and trust during this pregnancy and child's birth, we are thankful that You have put angels at watch over us and our child. We cast all the cares and burdens of this pregnancy to You. Father, Your Word declares that our unborn child was created in Your image, fearfully and wonderfully made. Thank You, Father, that all decisions regarding this pregnancy and delivery will be guided by the Holy Spirit.

In the name of Jesus Christ we cover my womb with the precious blood of Jesus Christ. Every good and perfect gift comes from You. I thank You, Father, that the baby already formed is Your workmanship, created in true perfection according to Your power. Father, all Your works are beautiful and magnificent to behold.

We cover the baby with the precious blood of Jesus. Your word says You made (insert name) and all the delicate inner parts of his/her body, knitting them together. You were there when (insert name) was formed, and right now You are still knitting him/her together, readying him/her to enter the world. In Jesus' name, amen.

A Prayer for After Tragedy

Abba, Father, we lift those experiencing tragedy into Your presence. We know that You will not let them face their battles alone, You will not in any way fail them or leave them without support. You will not leave them helpless or forsake them, nor let them down nor relax Your hold on them, assuredly not. But, indeed, You will come to them.

We pray, God, You would soothe them in this time of pain and grief, that You would ease the pain and sorrow, bring them relief, and console and encourage them. We pray the Holy Spirit would soothe them tenderly.

Lord, lift their spirits, drive away all despair, and flood their souls with Your love. We pray Your loving arms would hold them in Your embrace with the assurance that You will see them through. In Jesus' name, amen.

9

Conclusion

My heart, hope, and prayer is that after meeting all these beautiful woman, your sisters, and encountering their journeys, you feel inspired, encouraged, and filled with hope. Whatever you are facing, do not give up—keep going. Your miracle is right around the corner. Remember, you are not alone.

The necklace is symbolic of our faith; it reminds us that God is always working behind the scenes. Hebrews 11:1 says, "Faith is the confidence that what we hope for will actually happen, it gives us assurance about things we cannot see."

The other day my mom said, "Honey, I was thinking about something while I was doing my puzzle. Our journeys . . . our lives are unique, just like a puzzle. She went on in more detail. Every puzzle is made up of unique pieces and each piece of a puzzle has a perfect spot. Sometimes, we try to put those pieces in the wrong place. It may squeeze into place, but we know, ultimately, it's not quite right. So we have to take our time and put each piece where it goes, and then it all forms together to make a beautiful picture.

I thought to myself, "Wow, Mom, that's so good!" She is right; we are a piece of art created by the supreme Artist. We are His masterpiece, and each of our journeys is filled with numerous seasons or pieces of the puzzle, some warm and flourishing like a palm tree glistening in the sun and others frigid like a dark winter day.

But no matter what season of life we are in or what piece of the puzzle doesn't feel quite right, know that God already has the perfect design, the perfect plan. Sometimes the hardest part is being patient and waiting on Him.

Homeschooling my kids has taught us that patience is key to success! If you were to ask them what patience means, they would say, "Waiting without complaining!" Let's choose to live our lives with patience, not with complaints.

Ecclesiastes 3:1–15 says:

> *"For everything there is a season,*
> *a time for every activity under heaven.*
> *A time to be born and a time to die.*

A time to plant and a time to harvest.
A time to kill and a time to heal.
A time to tear down and a time to build up.
A time to cry and a time to laugh.
A time to grieve and a time to dance.
A time to scatter stones and a time to gather stones.
A time to embrace and a time to turn away.
A time to search and a time to quit searching.
A time to keep and a time to throw away.
A time to tear and a time to mend.
A time to be quiet and a time to speak.
A time to love and a time to hate.
A time for war and a time for peace.

What do people really get for all their hard work? I have seen the burden God has placed on many of us. Yet God has made everything beautiful in its own time. He has planted eternity in the human heart, but even so, people cannot see the whole scope of God's work from beginning to end. So I concluded there is nothing better than to be happy and enjoy ourselves as long as we can. And people should eat and drink and enjoy the fruits of their labors, for these are gifts from God.

And I know that whatever God does is final. Nothing can be added to it or taken from it. God's purpose is that people should fear Him. What is happening now has happened before, and what will happen in the future has happened before because God makes the same things happen over and over again.

As we journey through life's seasons I always remember that it is how we respond to what is happening to us that sets us apart. We cannot always choose the cards we are dealt, but we can choose how we will play them. Although this book is full of encouragement it does not disregard the pain, frustration, or stress that we all face. When you feel lost and broken, what you need and desire most is tenderness and support. That is what I hope you received when reading and sharing this book. We do not always have the answers, but we can put our trust in the One who does. God knows the beginning from the end, and His plan is far greater than we can ever fathom.

Jeremiah 29:11 says, "For I know the plans I have for you, declares the Lord, plans to prosper you and not harm you, plans to give you hope and a future." Take a deep breathe and know that with God your future is bright!

Another wonderful healing tool for the soul is laughter, the kind of laughter that brings tears of joy to your eyes and twinges to your belly! If you ask my family, they will tell you how much we love to laugh and find humor in everything we can! For instance, on days that I'm feeling sad or not quite myself, I turn the music on, open the windows, and sing as loud as I can. I love when the bass hits hard and I can feel the lyrics flowing through my body. That's when the kids start laughing like crazy. Or maybe its Mommy's dance moves. Either way we are all filled with joy, and it makes it easier to move forward in good spirits. If you are feeling conquered or it's simply just too hard to put one foot in front of the other, take my sweet mom's advice. Mama Marcia, as she is called by many, says, "Honey, just take it one day at a time!" If we put too much pressure on ourselves we can get lost in our despair and give up on our dreams and let our circumstances steal our joy.

Proverbs 13:12 (NLT) says, "Hope deferred makes the heart sick, but a dream fulfilled is a tree of life." The necklace really did take on a life of its own, branching out around the world. Each worn by a woman facing every day with living, breathing faith. A reminder hanging around their necks or incubators that with God all things are possible.

God is the one who made unbreakable covenants. In Him, we have promises the world can never offer. If you seek Him you will find Him and a life filled with purpose and hope. Lets keep the journey of the necklace alive.

Sisterhood, I pray that the Lord would shine his face upon you and wrap you up in His loving arms. May you always feel His holy and mighty presence and ultimately allow Him to be the true architect of your life.

Next Steps

Thank you for taking the journey with us!

After reading all these beautiful stories, I am sure God put someone on your heart who needs this book, a necklace, or the Sisterhood. Please do not ignore that still, small voice.

Continue the journey on our website to read updates, see pictures, get free resources, and more:

www.TheNecklaceBook.com/NextSteps

We would love it if you would do the following:

- Connect with us on our social networking site www.TheSocialNecklace.com
- Write a review of the book and share your thoughts with the world.
- Buy merchandise and help support the cause.

- Share a necklace and book with someone who needs it.
- Check out our doctor recommended health resources for fertility health.
- Start a necklace small group and bring hope to those on the journey.
- Attend or schedule a "necklace" event in your area.
- Share your fertility story with us.

About The Author

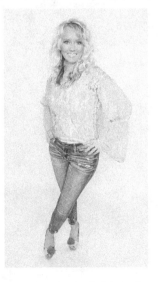

Nicole Wood has her Master's Degree in Pastoral Counseling. She is a solution-focused counselor and the founder of the Rockn Relationship movement, which helps couples experience the most satisfying relationship possible. She has worked with all types of couples, including celebrities, helping them get to the core of their issues.

Nicole and her husband, Joe, serve at FaithChurch. com in West Palm Beach Florida. They have been rockn their marriage since 2009 and have four beautiful children. Nicole enjoys spending lots of time on the beach, running marathons, fishing on tranquil mountain rivers, and encouraging people to believe God for the "impossible."

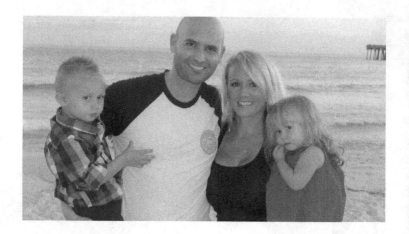

A free ebook edition is available with the purchase of this book.

To claim your free ebook edition:

1. Visit MorganJamesBOGO.com
2. Sign your name CLEARLY in the space
3. Complete the form and submit a photo of the entire copyright page
4. You or your friend can download the ebook to your preferred device

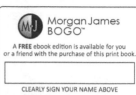

Morgan James BOGO™

A **FREE** ebook edition is available for you or a friend with the purchase of this print book.

CLEARLY SIGN YOUR NAME ABOVE

Instructions to claim your free ebook edition:
1. Visit MorganJamesBOGO.com
2. Sign your name CLEARLY in the space above
3. Complete the form and submit a photo of this entire page
4. You or your friend can download the ebook to your preferred device

Print & Digital Together Forever.

Snap a photo

Free ebook

Read anywhere

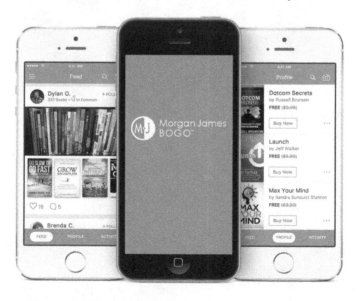

CPSIA information can be obtained
at www.ICGtesting.com
Printed in the USA
JSHW020218200821
18006JS00001B/30